Multiple Choice Questions

related to the

OXFORD TEXTBOOK OF MEDICINE

SECOND EDITION

Prepared by a panel of London consultant physicians

Edited by: Carol A Quarini MSc

Multiple Choice Questions
related to the
OXFORD TEXTBOOK OF MEDICINE
SECOND EDITION

Prepared by a panel of London consultant physicians

Edited by: Carol A Quarini MSc

PASTEST SERVICE
HEMEL HEMPSTEAD
HERTFORDSHIRE
ENGLAND

304 Galley Hill,
Hemel Hempstead, Hertfordshire.

First published 1983
Second edition 1987

British Library Cataloguing in Publication Data

Quarini, C.
MCQs related to the Oxford textbook of medicine, second series.
1. Medicine — Problems, exercises, etc.
I. Title
610'.76 R834.5

ISBN 0 906896 22 3

Text prepared by Turner Associates, Knutsford, Cheshire.
Phototypeset by Communitype, Leicester.
Printed by Biddles Ltd., Guildford, Surrey.

CONTENTS

Each section listed below contains questions based on the corresponding section in the Oxford Textbook of Medicine, second edition.

Note: brackets indicate the number of questions in each section.

INTRODUCTION

This PASTEST revision book contains 400 multiple choice questions related to the Oxford Textbook of Medicine, Oxford University Press, second edition 1987 edited by D. J. Weatherall, J. G. C. Ledingham, and D. A. Warrel. The questions cover all 25 main subject headings.

Each question consists of an initial statement (or 'stem') followed by five possible completions (or 'items') identified by ABCDE. There is no restriction on the number of true or false items in a question. It is possible for all the items in a question to be true, or for all to be false.

The answers to each question are to be found at the end of this book together with a specific page reference to the Oxford Textbook of Medicine, second edition. The student, having studied and answered the multiple choice questions in one section, can then check his answers and learn from his mistakes by turning to the specific pages referred to in the Oxford Textbook of Medicine. In this way a systematic method of revision can be achieved without attempting the daunting task of reading an entire section at a time!

The Oxford Textbook of Medicine, designed for students, trainees and specialists in internal medicine replaced Price's Textbook of Medicine as the major British textbook. A total of 283 internationally distinguished specialists were brought together and have produced a truly authoritative and comprehensive textbook.

Every effort has been made to ensure that the Oxford Textbook of Medicine is of value, not only to physicians practising in developed countries, but also to those in other parts of the world. For this reason there is extensive coverage of infectious and tropical diseases.

This PASTEST revision book will be an invaluable aid to students and specialists using the Oxford Textbook of Medicine. Prepared by specialists and edited by an expert in MCQs, this book will help them to check their knowledge of internal medicine.

SECTION 4: GENETICS

1. The following are correct statements concerning inheritance:

A in Britain the incidence of autosomal dominant disorders is about 7 per 1000 live births
B characters inherited as dominants are of varying seriousness in different individuals
C in autosomal recessive inheritance, if two homozygous subjects marry, all their children will be affected
D the distribution of height in a human population follows approximately a Gaussian curve
E hypertrophic pyloric stenosis is much commoner in girls than in boys

2. It is at present possible to make an antenatal diagnosis of

A sickle cell anaemia
B Huntington's chorea
C cystic fibrosis
D thalassaemia
E Down's syndrome

3. The following are examples of genetic polymorphism in man:

A rhesus blood groups
B white versus negro characteristics
C variation in blood pressure
D rate of acetylation of isoniazid
E glucose-6-phosphate dehydrogenase deficiency

4. The following chromosomal abnormalities give rise to the clinical conditions quoted:

A 47,XXX: abnormally tall stature
B 45,XO: Turner's syndrome
C 47, + 18: Down's syndrome
D 46,XY/47,XXY mosaic: Klinefelter's syndrome
E 45,5p-: cri du chat syndrome

5. The following hereditary disorders show an abnormally high predisposition to malignancy:

A xeroderma pigmentosum
B Bloom's syndrome
C Fanconi's anaemia
D ataxia talangiectasia
E cystinuria

6. The incidence of cancer of the organ mentioned is increased in the corresponding group:

A lip: pipe smokers
B large bowel: Ugandans
C liver: citizens of USA
D lung: inhabitants of capital cities
E pancreas: cigarette smokers

7. Basal-cell carcinoma of the skin

A accounts for the majority of cancers on the exposed skin
B is almost unknown in blacks
C is an important hazard of radiotherapy
D in the past has been common among chimney sweeps
E may be caused by prolonged exposure to arsenic

8. The incidence of carcinoma of the breast is increased in women who

A have an early menarche and late menopause
B take an oestrogen/progestogen oral contraceptive
C have their first child after the age of 35 years
D avoid breast feeding
E are nuns

9. Characteristic findings in the hyperviscosity syndrome include

A epistaxis
B congestive cardiac failure
C perforation of the nasal septum
D dilatation of retinal veins
E purpura on extensor aspects of distal areas of the limbs

10. The alkylating agents used in the chemotherapy of malignant disease

A are all teratogenic
B are all carcinogenic in experimental animals
C are not immunosuppressive
D cause amenorrhoea and flushing in women of child-bearing age
E are of particular value in the treatment of squamous-cell carcinoma of the bronchus

11. Methotrexate

A is poorly absorbed when given by mouth
B does not pass the blood-brain barrier
C is rapidly excreted unchanged by the kidneys
D is a purine analogue
E commonly causes haemorrhagic cystitis

SECTION 5: INFECTIONS

1. Infection with

A Schistosoma mansoni is more frequently severe in blood group A patients
B Plasmodium falciparum is commoner in subjects with haemoglobin genotype AS
C streptococci are less common in subjects with inherited complement deficiency
D malaria is less severe in adults
E yellow fever is milder in the young

2. The following primary infections predispose to the secondary infection quoted:

A influenza: bacterial pneumonia
B meningococcal disease: herpes zoster
C pneumococcal disease: aspergillosis
D septic abortion: gas gangrene
E malaria: salmonella septicaemia

3. In disinfection procedures

A Dettol is good at reducing the level of bacteria over a floor area
B Dettol destroys spores
C 20% formaldehyde in ethanol kills spores, bacteria and many viruses though it may take many hours
D glutaraldehyde 2% kills tubercle bacilli in ten minutes
E hexachlorophane is useful especially for children

4. The following statements constitute correct advice for travellers requiring immunisation:

A smallpox vaccination is now only required for a few African countries
B yellow fever vaccine can be given at the same time as oral polio vaccination
C typhoid vaccine can be given intradermally
D the only vaccinations required by international sanitary regulations are cholera and typhoid
E immunoglobulin for hepatitis A gives full protection against infection for at least 6 months

5. Travellers requiring advice about malaria prophylaxis should be told that

A daily proguanil is protective worldwide
B a combination of pyrimethamine and dapsone is useful
C chloroquine is the best prophylactic drug
D they must start one month before entering the endemic area
E they should continue for one week after returning home

6. The action of the following antimicrobial agents is as specified:

A penicillin works on the cell wall
B bacitracin inhibits peptidoglycan formation
C chloramphenicol interferes with messenger RNA translation
D erythromycin interferes with DNA
E metronidazole damages DNA

7. The following are recommended therapy for viral infections:

A amantadine for herpes simplex
B oral amantadine for influenza A
C topical idoxuridine (IDU) for herpes simplex
D intravenous acyclovir for severe herpes simplex
E intravenous vidarabine for herpes zoster in immuno- suppressed patients

8. The following clinical conditions may be caused by the respiratory viruses quoted:

A hand, foot and mouth disease: Cocksackie B virus
B glandular fever: Epstein-Barr virus
C croup in children: respiratory syncytial virus
D acute bronchiolitis: respiratory syncytial virus
E ulcerative pharyngitis: echovirus

9. Infection by herpes viruses in man

A may be caused by any one of at least nine distinct viruses
B is transmitted most readily in the case of Epstein-Barr virus
C requires close contact in the case of cytomegalovirus
D causing a whitlow should not be treated by incision
E is a particular hazard of Rugby football players

10. Chickenpox

A is commonly seen in a congenital form
B may be severe in a newborn child infected by the mother in late pregnancy
C affects the limbs more than the trunk
D may cause pneumonitis
E should be treated by intravenous vidarabine when there is evidence of hepatitis

11. Herpes zoster

A may commonly be reactivated by physical trauma to the affected dermatome
B is always painful
C is rarely seen in bilateral dermatomes
D of S2 dermatome may present as an acute retention of urine
E is found more often in patients with an underlying malignancy

12. Infectious mononucleosis

A is characterised by a monocytosis with at least 10% of atypical lymphocytes
B belongs to the same group of diseases as cytomegalovirus disease and toxoplasmosis and can be misdiagnosed as such
C is diagnosed by the heterophile agglutinins for sheep's red cells in the Paul-Bunnell test
D is diagnosed by the characteristic palatal petechiae rarely seen in any other disease
E causes a rise in EB specific IgM antibody which lasts for many months

13. Cytomegalovirus infections (CMV)

A cause large intranucleic inclusions
B cause infants to excrete the virus for months or even years
C cause hepato-splenomegaly in many congenital cases
D may be transmitted sexually
E give rise to a primary or reactivated infection in renal transplant patients

14. Pox viruses

A cause orf and molluscum contagiosum
B caused the last outbreak of endemic smallpox in 1977 in Somalia
C are best differentiated under the light microscope
D are endemic in gerbils
E are no longer a major threat to human life worldwide

15. Epidemic parotitis virus (mumps)

A can infect the liver, heart and joints
B has never been grown from breast milk
C cannot be reliably detected by means of antibody tests
D frequently invades the nervous system
E is an important cause of male sterility in Western society

16. In measles infections

A within the tropics, most cases are seen in the wet months
B in the temperate parts of the world, most cases occur in summer
C it is the antibody-antigen complex that causes the striking irritability of the child
D about 1 child in a million develops subacute sclerosing panencephalitis (SSPE)
E Koplik spots are seen two days before any other manifestation

17. Rubella infection

A has little medical importance save its ability to produce congenital abnormalities when women are infected during pregnancy
B often causes enlarged cervical and occipital lymph nodes
C in pregnant women may lead to Gregg's triad of cardiovascular defects, eye defects and deafness in the baby
D may be prevented by vaccination with a killed virus
E will be greatly reduced by the policy of vaccination of all 11-14- year-old children

18. Diseases caused by enteroviruses include

A Lassa fever
B Bornholm disease
C aseptic meningitis
D croup
E pericarditis

19. Rabies

A is endemic in Australia and New Zealand
B causes as many as 15,000 deaths annually in India alone
C has an incubation period of not less than two months
D causes death in 30% within a few days of the onset of hydrophobia
E can be distinguished from 'hydrophobic tetanus' by a longer incubation and the lack of trismus

20. Yellow fever

A was first recorded in Africa during the 18th century
B is transmitted by the Aedes aegypti mosquito
C is still the most important cause of viral haemorrhagic disease in Africa
D is characterised by jaundice in the early stages of the disease
E vaccination confers long-lasting immunity

21. Lassa fever

A has been known in North Nigeria for over a century
B occurs in Africa only in epidemic form
C is easy to diagnose clinically as it has such a sudden onset of coughing
D can only be brought to Europe by travellers from West Africa
E requires isolation nursing

22. Hepatitis A

A has an incubation period usually between three and five weeks
B is not transmitted by blood or blood products
C is characterised by parenchymal liver cell necrosis and histiocytic periportal inflammation
D virus has not yet been isolated
E cannot at present be propagated in cell culture

23. Hepatitis B

A virus has a surface antigen often referred to as Australia antigen
B has a shorter incubation period than hepatitis A
C may be transmitted by sexual contact
D may play a part in the aetiology of liver cell carcinoma
E causes a persistent carrier state in children infected during the perinatal period

24. In associating human disease with tumour viruses it has been shown that

A Epstein-Barr virus is associated with Burkitt's lymphoma
B Epstein-Barr virus is associated with naso-pharyngeal carcinoma
C cytomegalovirus antigens are seen in Kaposi's sarcoma cells
D folyoma JC virus is associated with progressive multifocal leucoencephalopathy
E SV40 viruses may cause malignant melanoma

25. The following are correct statements about diphtheria:

A the causal organism is a Gram-negative bacterium
B strains of the organism are best tested for toxin production by radioimmunoassay
C the Schick test is a measure of susceptibility to the disease
D in laryngeal diphtheria there is often no membrane on the throat at all
E the disease can be prevented with absolute certainty if appropriate immunisation is given

26. Scarlet fever

A is caused by the erythrogenic toxin of group A streptococci
B is no longer a notifiable disease
C has a specific clinical sign seen in no other condition, circumoral pallor
D may cause intense itching
E causes the tongue to be furred with red-tipped papillae

27. The following are major criteria in the Jones system for the diagnosis of rheumatic fever:

A erythema marginatum
B positive test for C-reactive protein
C prolonged P-R interval in the electrocardiogram
D subcutaneous nodules
E arthralgia

28. Pneumococcal infections

A are caused by some 83 different serotypes as seen in the quellung reaction
B are a common cause of otitis media in young children
C as seen in lobarn pneumonia allow complete anatomical and functional recovery
D do not produce a bronchopneumonia
E may cause peritonitis in young healthy girls

29. Staphylococcus aureus

A produces at least six enterotoxins responsible for food poisoning
B enterotoxins cause vomiting and diarrhoea one to six hours after ingestion
C is responsible for pemphigus neonatorum and sycosis barbae
D gives rise to hordeola
E food poisoning is best treated by anti-bacterial chemotherapy

30. Staphylococcus aureus

A phage group 1 has been implicated as the cause of toxic-shock syndrome in children
B is thought to be the cause of toxic-shock syndrome seen in menstruating women using internal tampons
C is a common cause of subacute bacterial endocarditis
D is an important cause of endocarditis after intra-cardiac prosthetic surgery
E is the commonest cause of osteomyelitis at all ages

31. Meningococcal infection

A is caused by bean-shaped, Gram-positive diplococci
B is seen only in temperate climates
C is reported in the UK about 100-200 times a year
D produces clinical disease in 80% of cases
E clinically has the features of an acute endotoxaemia

32. In the diagnosis and treatment of acute meningococcaemia

A there may be leucopenia in the peripheral blood
B the respiratory rate is usually decreased
C consciousness is not impaired unless the blood pressure falls
D the best drug is crystalline penicillin
E the best drug to use for penicillin sensitive people is cloramphenicol

33. Salmonella infections

A are caused by lactose fermenting members of the Enterobacteriaceae family
B are caused by some 2000 serotypes
C in Britain are most commonly due to S. typhimurium
D may cause bloody diarrhoea
E can be dangerous in maternity units

34. Salmonella

A food poisoning is caused by the toxins produced during cooking
B infection is increased in those using antacids
C infection may present clinically up to 2 days post infection
D osteomyelitis is strongly associated with sickle-cell anaemia
E enteritis is best treated by ampicillin therapy

35. Bacillary dysentery

A may be caused by Shigella sonnei
B is caused by four groups of bacilli which are differentiated by their biochemical reactions and antigenic structure
C requires a larger infective dose than salmonella infection
D is often transmitted by flies
E may be helped by purgation to clear the bowel of toxins

36. Infantile gastroenteritis caused by Escherichia coli (EPEC)

A in the tropics is commonest among new-born babies
B may cause death in babies whose bowel is essentially normal at post-mortem
C may have an incubation period of only eight hours
D should be treated vigorously with antibiotics
E should be treated by rehydration

37. Enterotoxigenic E. coli (ETEC)

A are very common in temperate zones
B may cause water-borne epidemics
C may cause outbreaks of meningitis on cruise ships
D produce a toxin which increases the production of adenyl cyclase
E is best treated by low doses of Enterovioform

38. Campylobacters

A have a single flagellum at each end
B are found in the normal intestinal flora of birds
C are the commonest bacterial pathogens isolated from patients with acute enterocolitis
D are easily typed and therefore make source tracing a simple procedure
E causing enterocolitis in families are nearly always acquired from a new puppy or kitten

39. Typhoid fever

A invariably comes originally from a human source
B may be contracted from shellfish
C is caused by bacilli which multiply in the duodenum
D is easily diagnosed by blood culture in the third or fourth week
E may cause lesions of Peyer's patches

40. Typhoid fever

A has a characteristic macular rash with rose spots
B is a common cause of acute cholecystitis in the developing world
C may be diagnosed by positive stool cultures during the third week of the illness
D is diagnosed by measuring antibody titre to flagellar (H) and somatic (O) antigens
E causes leucopenia only in a small minority of patients

41. Anaerobic infections

A include Vincent's angina
B are almost all sensitive to metronidazole
C are resistant to chloramphenicol
D are usually sensitive to tetracycline
E due to Clostridium perfringens (welchii) are sensitve to ampicillin

42. Cholera

A immunisation provides 100% protection for three months in endemic areas
B has been endemic in the Ganges Delta for over 200 years
C does not affect any other species but man
D susceptibility is decreased following a subtotal gastrectomy
E should not be treated by the use of antimicrobials

43. Haemophilus influenzae

A is commonly carried in the nasopharynx of healthy people and may be regarded as normal flora
B is the commonest cause of bacterial meningitis in children below the age of five
C may give rise to a clinical condition similar to meningococcal infection including the Waterhouse-Friderichsen syndrome
D is best treated by chloramphenicol if the cause of a severe infection
E may cause epiglottitis which is best diagnosed by the G.P. on direct examination

44. Bordetella pertussis

A is found in many domestic animals
B causes ciliostasis and eventual loss of ciliated cells
C is often carried by clinically healthy subjects
D can be recovered from the blood in cases of whooping-cough
E immunity produced by bacterial vaccine is life long

45. Plague

A is caused by Yersinia pestis a small ovoid bacillus which is non-sporing
B is transmitted among animals by fleas
C is found in the wild in large areas of the USA
D buboes should be surgically drained whenever possible
E responds well to high doses of penicillin

46. Bacillus anthracis

A is a Gram-negative, motile organism
B forms spores very readily in anaerobic conditions
C is primarily the causative agent of a disease of cattle, sheep and goats with a very high mortality in these animals
D may be contracted by the handling of ivory
E causes sores with a coal-black centre which are best treated by tetracycline

47. Brucellosis

A constitutes an increased risk to patients with achlorhydria
B may be transmitted sexually or following blood transfusion
C is thought to cause no more abortions or miscarriages than any other severe acute infection
D is rare in children
E is best treated by a long course of tetracyclines and streptomycin

48. Tetanus

A is caused by a Gram-positive bacillus which will only grow in anaerobic conditions
B has approximately 50% mortality worldwide
C bacillus toxin may pass along sympathetic nerve fibres causing overactivity
D always causes muscular rigidity
E confers life-long immunity

49. Tuberculosis

A is caused by Mycobacterium tuberculosis which is capable of either intracellular or extracellular existence
B vaccine BCG is a form of M. bovis
C in Indian immigrants to the UK is usually caused by Indian strains of the organism
D produces its clinical effects by the actions of exotoxins and extracellular enzymes from the tubercle bacillus
E can be very reliably diagnosed by laryngeal swabs

50. Tuberculosis

A resistance to rifampicin and ethambutol is now commonplace
B nearly always causes those infected to become clinically ill
C among Eskimos often occurs in a fulminating form
D testing with the Mantoux test should be performed strictly subcutaneously
E vaccination with BCG often causes severe adverse reactions

51. Leprosy

A bacilli are widespread in lesions of the tuberculoid form of the disease
B has a large animal reservoir
C bacilli are engulfed by Schwann cells
D in untreated lactating mothers may be passed on through the breast milk
E may present in children as areas of hyperpigmentation

52. Syphilis

A has an infectivity of about 2% after a single exposure
B in its congenital form is seen in 200 cases a year in the UK
C has recently had an increased rate of infection due to ‘the pill’
D seen as a gumma is now rare
E in the secondary stage usually causes considerable constitutional disturbance

53. In the detection and diagnosis of syphilis

A the rapid plasma reagin (RPR) test is no longer useful for screening purposes
B the VDRL test is a qualitative but not a quantitative test
C the VDRL is most useful in detecting re-infection due to a sustained rise of titre
D the T. pallidum immobilization (TPI) test uses live treponemes
E biological false-positive tests may be caused by mycoplasma pneumonia

54. The Leptospira interrogans complex

A causes a disease in rodents which is usually fatal
B mostly affects the kidney and liver
C causes a rise in IgM antibodies which disappears after the first week of the disease
D causes primarily vascular changes
E can be prevented by an effective vaccine which is used worldwide

55. Cat scratch disease is

A associated with positive Frei skin test
B caused by a DNA virus
C associated with a pathognomonic histological picture
D associated with regional lymphadenopathy
E associated with a positive Hangar-Rose test

56. Tetracycline can be used to treat

A Whipple's disease
B chancroid
C yaws
D granuloma inguinale
E non gonococcal urethritis

57. Chlamydia trachomatis has been implicated as a causal agent in

A pelvic inflammatory disease
B granuloma inguinale
C psittacosis
D Curtis-Fitz Hugh syndrome
E rhinosporidiosis

58. The following statements are true:

A TPHA and FTA tests can differentiate between yaws and syphilis
B yaws is transmitted venereally
C yaws is caused by Treponema carteum
D bejel is caused by Treponema pallidum
E infections with Treponema carteum only affect the skin

59. Painful genital ulcers occur in

A primary syphilis
B Herpes genitalis
C lympho-granuloma venereum
D Granuloma inguinale
E chancroid

60. In infections with Neisseria gonorrhoeae

A the squamous epithelium is infected
B urethral strictures are a common complication
C homosexuals are always symptomatic
D pelvic inflammatory disease occurs in 10-15% of untreated women
E resistance to penicillin is always due to penicillinase production

61. Cell culture systems can be used to isolate

A Chlamydia trachomatis
B Chlamydia psittaci
C Sarcocystis hominis
D Rickettsia
E Bartonella bacilliformis

62. The following infections are transmitted to man by tick bites:

A Q fever
B Rocky Mountain spotted fever
C Rickettsial pox
D Bartonellosis
E Scrub typhus

63. The following organisms are found in infections caused by bites:

A Eikenella corrodens
B Haemophilus aphophilus
C DF-2
D Arachnia propionica
E Pasteurella multocida

64. Reiter's disease

A is most commonly found in young men aged between 20-30 years
B can follow salmonella infections
C can be associated with meningoencephalitis
D occurs once only
E is always associated with ankylosing spondylitis

65. An incubation period of 2-4 days occurs in

A Herpes genitalis
B Brill-Zinsser disease
C Q fever
D chlamydial urethritis
E yaws

66. Pneumonia can be caused by the following organisms:

A Chlamydia psittaci
B Chlamydia trachomatis
C Mycoplasma orale
D Toxoplasma gondii
E Echinococcus granulosus

67. After eating poorly cooked meat, humans can become infected with the following organisms:

A Trichinella spiralis
B Enterobius vermicularis
C Trichuris trichiura
D Gnathostoma spinigerum
E Taenia saginata

68. The following organisms can cause systemic infections:

A Histoplasma capsulatum
B Malassezia furfur
C Leishmania mexicana
D Babesia microti
E Echinococcus granulosus

69. Common clinical features of Reiter's disease are

A urethritis
B aortic incompetence
C polyarthritis
D keratitis
E hepatitis

70. The following are characteristics of mycoplasma:

A it contains RNA and DNA
B its multiplication is dependent on host cell nucleic acid
C it is sensitive to cell wall antibiotics
D its growth is inhibited by a specific antibody
E it cannot multiply on a cell free medium

71. The following organisms can cause mycetomas:

A Nocardia asteroides
B Actinomadura madurae
C Madurella mycetomatis
D Sporothrix schenckii
E Candida parapsilosis

72. Systemic fungal infections can be caused by the following:

A Cryptococcus neoformans
B Histoplasma capsulatum
C Paracoccidioides brasiliensis
D Naegleria fowleri
E Isospora belli

73. Thiabendazole is effective in eliminating

A Strongyloides stercoralis
B Ancylostoma duodenale
C Necator americanus
D Trichinella spiralis
E Enterobius vermicularis

74. Transplacental infections can occur with the following:

A N. gonorrhoea
B Treponema pallidum
C Toxoplasma gondii
D Pseudomonas aeruginosa
E Coxsackie B virus

75. In human pediculosis

A the causative organism is Sarcoptes scabei
B a blepharoconjunctivitis may occur
C head shaving is not necessary for treatment
D clothes must be burnt to destroy the lice
E infection does not spread within the family

76. Non gonococcal urethritis

A is always caused by Chlamydia trachomatis
B can have an incubation period of 2 months
C can recur after treatment
D can be differentiated clinically from gonorrhoea
E may respond to co-trimoxazole

77. Metronidazole can be used to treat infections caused by

A Gardnerella vaginalis
B Listeria monocytogenes
C E. histolytica
D Naegleria fowleri
E Trichomonas vaginalis

SECTION 6: CHEMICAL AND PHYSICAL INJURIES, CLIMATIC AND OCCUPATIONAL DISEASES

1. The following industrial materials are known to have a toxic effect on the central nervous system:

A asbestos
B lead
C cadmium
D organo-phosphorus insecticides
E mercury

2. Angiosarcoma of the liver is a form of occupational cancer associated with exposure to

A beryllium
B crocidolite
C vinyl chloride
D toluene di-isocyanate
E organo-tin

3. Eye damage may be caused by the following agents:

A high voltage electric currents
B deep sea diving
C ipomoea (Morning Glory)
D methanol
E vibration

4. Specific antidotes exist for poisoning by

A cyanides
B aspirin
C organo-phosphorus compounds
D phenol
E barbiturates

5. Pulmonary oedema is a hazard associated with

A immersion hypothermia
B ozone poisoning
C radiation sickness
D acute mountain sickness
E snake bite

6. Methaemoglobinaemia may result from exposure to

A carbon monoxide
B isopropyl alcohol
C aniline
D trichlorethylene
E sodium chlorate

7. Toxic chemicals and drugs causing damage to renal tubules and glomeruli include

A cadmium
B antihistamines
C kerosene
D mercury
E epoxy resins

8. Which of the following drugs should *not* be administered to airline pilots on flying duties:

A diazepam
B tetracycline
C penicillin
D maloprim
E streptomycin

9. The following materials are known to cause occupational asthma:

A arsenic compounds
B isocyanates
C trimellitic acid anhydride
D carbon tetrachloride
E chloroplatinates

10. Chronic benzene poisoning is both a notifiable and a prescribed industrial disease. It causes

A aplastic anaemia
B extrinsic allergic alveolitis
C hepatic cirrhosis
D leukaemia
E renal tubular dysfunction

11. Liver damage is an important feature of chronic poisoning by

A carbon monoxide
B carbon tetrachloride
C carbon disulphide
D ethylene glycol
E nitrobenzene

12. In recent years a large number of substances have come under suspicion as occupational carcinogens. The following are now generally accepted as causing human cancer:

A kaolin
B benzidine
C nicotine
D arsenic
E nickel compounds

13. Notifiable industrial diseases which by statute must be reported to the Chief Employment Medical Adviser include:

A manganese poisoning
B farmers' lung
C anthrax
D toxic jaundice
E compressed air illness

SECTION 7: CLINICAL PHARMACOLOGY

1. When two related drugs are compared, one with high and the other with low lipid solubility, it is to be expected that the former will be

A better absorbed from the gut
B excreted unchanged more rapidly by the kidney
C more rapidly metabolised by the liver
D more likely to cause side-effects in the central nervous system
E more likely to cause B adverse reactions

2. Drug metabolism is increased by

A heavy smoking of cigarettes
B low protein, high carbohydrate diets
C severe malnutrition
D administration of allopurinol
E administration of rifampicin

SECTION 8: NUTRITION

1. The utilisation of a given energy-containing substrate by a tissue

A is related to its circulating concentration
B is related to the blood flow to the tissue
C is not related to blood flow to other tissues
D is not influenced by other substrates
E depends on certain characteristics of the plasma membrane

2. The following hormones play a catabolic rather than an anabolic role in metabolism:

A catecholamines
B insulin
C glucagon
D cortisol
E lipase

3. The short-term metabolic effects of insulin include

A increased glucose transport to the liver
B increased glucose transport to muscle
C increased gluconeogenesis
D increased glycogen synthesis
E decreased lipolysis

4. Apart from famine conditions, protein energy malnutrition may be secondary to

A infection
B anorexia nervosa
C malabsorption syndrome
D malignancy
E certain forms of cardiac disease

5. The clinical features of kwashiorkor include

A increased growth of eyebrow hair
B oedema
C desquamated skin
D fine friable discoloured hair
E decrease in liver size

6. Malnutrition may be classified according to

A Gomez classification, characterising the child according to the relation of weight to that of other children
B Wellcome system of classification according to weight deficit and presence or absence of oedema
C Waterlow classification based on height alone
D upper arm circumference
E Metropolitan Life Assurance tables of ideal weight for height

7. Mortality is increased by excess weight in men suffering from

A diabetes mellitus
B cerebral vascular disease
C hypertensive heart disease
D hypoventilation syndrome
E gall bladder disease

8. Characteristic signs of vitamin A deficiency include

A tenderness of legs
B bleeding at site of erupting teeth
C dryness of the conjunctiva
D Bitot's spots
E keratomalacia

9. Symptoms of hypervitaminosis A include

A impaired dark adaptation
B headache
C vomiting
D peeling of skin
E impaired cell-mediated immunity

10. Deficiency of thiamin (vitamin B_1) leads to

A loss of tendon reflexes
B muscle atrophy
C toe drop
D dyssebacea (shark skin)
E cheilosis (fissuring of vermilion surfaces of lips)

11. Among the trace elements essential for man are

A manganese
B chromium
C selenium
D molybdenum
E barium

12. Practicable methods of measuring body fat content are

A measurement of total body water
B measurement of total body potassium
C total body density
D uptake of fat soluble gas by the body
E skinfold thickness

13. Some complications of enteral feeding are

A oesophagitis resulting from tube insertion
B constipation
C elevated circulating concentrations of potassium and phosphate
D hyperglycaemia
E deficiency of fatty acids

14. Features of anorexia nervosa include

A bradycardia
B faulty perception of body size
C low oestrogen concentrations
D elevated LH and FSH concentrations
E excess of downy hair

SECTION 9: METABOLIC DISORDERS

1. The following are correct statements within the framework of the modern classification of diabetes mellitus:

A Type I diabetes can present at any age
B persistent islet-cell antibodies can be demonstrated in all Type I patients
C Type I patients eventually lose the power to secrete insulin
D obese Type II patients have raised insulin levels
E ketoacidosis does not occur in Type II diabetes

2. The secretion of insulin is stimulated by

A ß-adrenergic agents
B glucagon
C sympathetic nerve stimulation
D leucine
E somatostatin

3. The metabolic effects of insulin include promotion of

A glycogenesis in liver and muscle
B glycolysis in liver and muscle
C fatty acid oxidation in muscle
D urea production in liver
E phosphate entry into muscle

4. Dietary treatment of diabetes should be guided by the following principles:

A carbohydrates should supply about half the total calories
B simple sugars are permissible provided the carbohydrate ration is not exceeded
C food intake should be well spread out throughout the day
D snacks between the main meals and at night should be forbidden
E the fat intake should contain as high a proportion of polyunsaturated fatty acids as possible

5. Sulphonylurea drugs

A act by increasing the response of pancreatic ß-cells to a given level of glucose
B have no extra-pancreatic action
C are particularly effective when given in conjunction with insulin
D can all cause hypoglycaemia
E are liable to cause lactic acidosis

6. Human insulin

A is closer to porcine than to bovine insulin in molecular structure
B is now available commercially
C is 2.5 times more effective, weight for weight, than porcine insulin
D is thought to be more rapidly absorbed from the injection site than porcine insulin
E is particularly liable to cause fat atrophy at injection sites

7. Factors increasing the rate of absorption of insulin after subcutaneous injection include

A use of acid rather than neutral preparations
B use of concentrated insulin preparations
C injection under the skin of the abdomen compared with the thigh
D deep rather than shallow s.c. injection
E massage of the site

8. Insulins suitable for intravenous injection include

A isophane
B hypurin neutral
C neusulin
D monotard
E neuphane

9. Measurement of glycosylated haemoglobin

A is best carried out by immunoassay
B gives an integrated assessment of the control blood glucose levels over several weeks
C gives results which are independent of red-cell life span
D requires preliminary dialysis or incubation in saline
E is not adaptable to auto-analytical machines

10. In patients with known or possible diabetic retinopathy

A mydriatics should be avoided in retinoscopy because of the risk of precipitating open-angle glaucoma
B retinoscopic review should be carried out annually in all diagnosed over the age of 40
C proliferative change is more likely in younger patients
D spontaneous arrest of deterioration of retinopathy is unknown
E once retinitis proliferans has become established, treatment has no effect

11. The following responses to infection are known to be impaired in poorly controlled diabetics:

A chemotaxis of polymorph leucocytes
B phagocytosis
C production of the C4 component of complement
D production of opsonins
E microbicidal activity of polymorph leucocytes

12. In severe diabetic ketoacidosis

A potassium should be given as soon as saline and insulin infusion have been started
B potassium requirements are likely to be higher in newly diagnosed than in known diabetics
C bicarbonate infusion should be started as soon as possible
D hypotonic rather than isotonic saline infusion should be given
E insulin should not be given subcutaneously

13. Chylomicrons

A are transported by pinocytosis from the intestinal lumen to the blood stream
B are not normally present in fasting plasma
C are rich in triglyceride
D are initially metabolised in peripheral tissues
E impart lactescence to the plasma if present in large numbers

14. In the treatment of acute gouty arthritis

A salicylates should not be used
B allopurinol should be given from the outset
C if there is no response to appropriate therapy within 48 hours the diagnosis should be reviewed
D diuretics should be avoided if possible
E if hydrocortisone is given there is a risk of toxic epidermal necrolysis

15. Characteristic findings in cutaneous hepatic porphyria include

A severe abdominal pain with vomiting
B a history of excessive alcohol consumption
C symmetrical peripheral neuropathy
D hirsutism in women
E raised urinary porphobilinogen

16. In Wilson's disease

A a Kayser-Fleischer ring is always present if the patient has neurological manifestations
B the most reliable diagnostic test is estimation of urinary copper excretion
C a mainstay of treatment is a diet low in copper
D patients who develop fever and urticaria when given penicillamine should never be given this drug again
E most patients will not respond to treatment in the first 6 months

17. The anion gap is increased in

A uraemic acidosis
B diabetic ketoacidosis
C classical renal tubular acidosis
D lactic acidosis
E methanol-induced acidosis

SECTION 10: ENDOCRINE DISORDERS

1. Growth hormone deficiency

A does not affect growth *in utero*
B in children is usually accompanied by delayed puberty
C is best demonstrated by measuring the GH response to a glucose tolerance test
D occurs early in the presentation of most pituitary diseases
E in adults may lead to hyperglycaemia

2. Elevation of the serum prolactin level may be caused by

A craniopharyngioma
B hyperthyroidism
C administration of oral contraceptives
D carcinoma of the bronchus
E administration of chlorpromazine

3. Failure or impairment of the response to TRH may be found in

A ophthalmic Graves' disease
B de Quervain's thyroiditis
C acromegaly
D Cushing's syndrome
E euthyroid multinodular goitre

4. In endemic goitre

A investigation invariably shows some degree of hypothyroidism
B there is clear evidence of an increased incidence of carcinoma of the thyroid
C administration of thyroxine will often cause the goitre to shrink
D administration of iodine occasionally precipitates hyperthyroidism
E the incidence after puberty is much higher in females

5. In hyperophthalmopathic Graves' disease

A one eye may be normal
B clinical evidence of hyperthyroidism is always present
C the finding of ophthalmoplegia suggests that myasthenia gravis is present as well
D oral corticosteroids are often beneficial
E spontaneous remissions and relapses are common

6. The following are correct statements about nodular goitre:

A a gland with multiple nodules is more likely to be malignant than one with a single nodule
B a single nodule which concentrates radio-iodine is very unlikely to be malignant
C if a 'cold' nodule can be shown by ultrasound to be cystic it is unlikely to be malignant
D 80% of multinodular goitres will regress on treatment with thyroxine
E in toxic nodular goitre, radio-iodine therapy is absolutely contraindicated

7. Papillary carcinoma of the thyroid

A is the commonest type of thyroid carcinoma
B carries the worst prognosis
C may secrete calcitonin
D should be treated by total thyroidectomy with radical neck dissection
E may metastasize to bone

8. In the medical management of hyperthyroidism

A the relapse rate after a full course of carbimazole is at least 50%
B if side-effects and toxic effects are not seen within two months of starting treatment with anti-thyroid drugs, then they may be regarded as extremely safe
C if agranulocytosis develops in a patient taking an anti-thyroid drug and this is withdrawn immediately, granulocytes may be expected to reappear within a few days
D beta adrenergic blocking drugs should not be given until the usual diagnostic tests have been completed
E the incidence of hypothyroidism 20 years after radio-iodine therapy may reach 50%

9. Calcitonin

A in normal humans is produced exclusively by the para-follicular cells of the thyroid
B reduces the number and activity of osteoclasts
C reduces renal tubular reabsorption of calcium
D reduces renal tubular reabsorption of phosphate
E if present in excess commonly causes tetany

10. In Cushing's syndrome

A muscular wasting affects proximal muscles more than distal ones
B more than half the patients are hypertensive at the time of diagnosis
C eosinophilia is common
D hypokalaemia is suggestive of a malignant cause
E if a pituitary micro-adenoma is the cause, its removal may be expected to restore normal ACTH function

11. In the investigation of Cushing's syndrome

A the best indicator of adrenocortical over-activity is a raised level of cortisol in a random sample of plasma
B a normal tomographic X-ray of the pituitary fossa rules out a pituitary cause
C dexamethasone suppression tests will distinguish accurately between Cushing's syndrome and obesity in 90-95% of cases
D plasma ACTH assay is valuable in defining an adrenal cause
E the metyrapone test helps to distinguish between an adrenal and a pituitary cause

12. Infertility

A due to abnormality in the male is usually amenable to treatment
B is associated with pathology of the Fallopian tubes in some 20% of couples
C due to varicocele responds to surgery in 30-50% of cases
D due to hyperprolactinaemia in the male responds well to bromocriptine
E due to tuberculous epididymitis is usually cured by anti-tuberculous therapy

13. In testicular feminization

A sex orientation is female
B the chromosome karyotype is 46XY
C testosterone is undetectable in the serum
D serum oestrogen levels are high at puberty
E the usual presentation in childhood is with inguinal herniae

14. Amenorrhoea with normal sex-hormone and gonadotrophin levels would be consistent with a diagnosis of

A polycystic ovary
B obesity
C Kallman's syndrome
D anorcxia
E ovarian dysgenesis

15. Recognised causes of hirsutism in women include

A congenital adrenal hyperplasia
B juvenile hypothyroidism
C secondary hypoadrenalism
D arrhenoblastoma of ovary
E treatment with diazoxide

SECTION 11: REPRODUCTIVE MEDICINE

1. The benefits of oral contraception include

A suppression of menstrual disorders
B suppression of functional ovarian cysts
C reduced incidence of gall bladder disease
D lessened risk of cancer of the ovary
E lessened risk of cancer of the breast

2. The risks of oral contraception include

A myocardial infarction
B hypotension
C hepatocellular adenoma
D cervical erosion
E impairment of fertility

3. The following oral anti-hypertensive agents may be used in pregnancy:

A reserpine
B bethanidine
C clonidine
D captopril
E prazosin

4. Acute renal failure in pregnancy

A is associated with low fetal mortality
B is commonly caused by abruptio placenti
C is caused by severe pre-eclampsia
D cannot be treated by peritoneal dialysis
E can be treated by haemodialysis

5. In the United Kingdom a commonly occurring heart disease in pregnancy is

A acute rheumatic carditis
B congenital heart disease
C peripartum cardiomyopathy
D myocardial infarction
E primary pulmonary hypertension

6. Insulin dependent diabetes adversely affects pregnancy; obstetric complications include

A pre-eclampsia
B polyhydramnios
C maternal infection
D fetal macrosomia
E congenital malformations

SECTION 12: GASTROENTEROLOGY

1. Pain from the

A oesophagus may radiate into the back
B colon is often poorly localised
C pancreas is relieved by lying flat
D stomach is transmitted up the vagus nerve
E small intestine is felt in the mid-line

2. Dental caries

A does not develop in the absence of cariogenic bacteria
B is promoted more effectively by glucose than by sucrose
C does not occur unless the pH at the enamel surface falls below about 5.5
D destroys enamel more rapidly than dentine
E is not prevented by using toothpaste containing fluoride

3. The following are correct statements about the migrating motor complex (MMC) of the gastrointestinal tract:

A activity in the lower oesophagus precedes that in the stomach by 15- 20 minutes
B during the activity front the stomach contracts about 3 times per minute
C the complex reaches the terminal ileum in about 100 minutes
D appearance of the MMC in the stomach is accompanied by increased gastric and pancreatic secretion
E the MMC does not traverse the colon

4. Gastro-oesophageal reflux

A may occur in the absence of hiatus hernia
B is rare in pregnancy
C is commonly relieved by weight reduction
D is associated with an increased incidence of oesophageal carcinoma
E responds better to H_2-receptor antagonists than to antacids

5. Achalasia

A is a painless condition
B causes dysphagia with fluids but not with solids
C is relieved by the administration of methacholine
D of long standing may lead to oesophageal carcinoma
E makes endoscopy of the stomach and duodenum impossible

6. Characteristic findings in the irritable bowel syndrome include

A abnormal sensitivity of the colon to vasoactive intestinal peptide
B diagnostic appearances in a barium enema X-ray
C normal or less than normal daily stool weight
D absence of blood in the stools
E normal blood sedimentation rate

7. Gastrin

A is released in response to protein ingestion
B is mainly found in the gastric antrum
C is released in large amounts during treatment with cimetidine
D is released in excessive amounts in patients with duodenal ulcer
E causes gastric pepsin secretion as its main action

8. In a patient in whom a pancreatic endocrine tumour has been demonstrated, the following additional investigations are essential:

A plasma calcium level
B plasma potassium level
C X-ray of the skull
D plasma calcitonin level
E urine vanillyl-mandelic acid output

9. In coeliac disease and tropical sprue a standard test breakfast produces unduly high plasma levels of

A enteroglucagon
B gastric inhibitory polypeptide
C motilin
D secretin
E gastrin

10. Gastric inhibitory polypeptide

A occurs mainly in the upper small intestine
B is released by ingestion of glucose
C is not released by ingestion of protein or fat
D causes secretion of insulin
E reduces gastric acid secretion

11. In the Zollinger-Ellison syndrome

A the fasting plasma gastrin is raised
B injection of secretin causes a fall in plasma gastrin
C injection of calcium salts causes an abnormal rise in plasma gastrin
D cimetidine gives symptomatic relief in many cases
E steatorrhoea may be a prominent feature

12. Recognised features of the carcinoid syndrome include

A precipitation of attacks by alcohol ingestion
B wheezing
C profuse diarrhoea
D pellagra
E improvement following removal of hepatic metastases

13. In the diagnosis of duodenal ulcer

A a firm diagnosis can be made from the history alone in 80-85% of cases
B the best diagnostic investigation is fibre-optic endoscopy
C the most suitable endoscope is the end-viewing type
D gastric secretory tests have no place
E plasma gastrin should be measured in patients with severe or ectopic ulceration

14. Acute erosive ulceration of the stomach or duodenum

A is a recognised sequel of head injury
B usually presents with haemorrhage
C can be prevented by giving H_2-blockers
D when established is immediately controlled by H_2-blockers
E responds well to surgery if medical treatment fails

15. In the management of upper gastrointestinal haemorrhage

A the risk of repeated haemorrhage is greatly reduced by giving H_2-blockers
B endoscopy carries definite morbidity and mortality risks
C endoscopy may allow identification of patients with a high risk of repeated haemorrhage
D a patient with a CVP of 0 cm or higher should not be transfused even if anaemic
E as a rough rule, one pack of blood will raise an adult patient's haemoglobin level by 1 g/dl

16. The following are correct statements regarding peptic ulceration:

A symptomatic relapse is firm evidence that a gastric or duodenal ulcer has recurred
B some 30% of recurrences in duodenal ulceration are symptomless
C there is clear evidence that giving up smoking hastens the healing of a duodenal ulcer
D antacids have no influence on the frequency of relapses
E antacid consumption is a good guide to the patient's progress

17. Treatment of peptic ulcer with cimetidine

A usually abolishes symptoms within 1 week
B produces healing in 70-80% of cases within 8 weeks
C may cause gynaecomastia
D carries a well-defined risk of gastric carcinoma in certain patients
E when discontinued is followed by rebound hyper-secretion of gastric acid

18. In primary hypogammaglobulinaemia there is an increased incidence of

A achlorhydria
B dental caries
C gastric carcinoma
D giardiasis
E nodular lymphoid hyperplasia of the small bowel

19. In the xylose absorption test, an abnormally low result could reasonably be explained by

A lymphoma of the small intestine
B chronic pancreatitis
C pyloric stenosis
D low urine flow
E renal failure

20. In the management of coeliac disease

A confirmation of the diagnosis in young children requires a total of three intestinal biopsies
B a faecal fat estimation is essential to confirm the diagnosis
C in adults a clinical response to a gluten-free diet may take up to a year to become manifest
D corticosteroid therapy involves a serious risk of intestinal perforation
E deterioration after a response to the diet should suggest a lymphoma of the small intestine

21. In tropical sprue

A diagnosis depends on demonstration of characteristic appearances in the intestinal biopsy
B vitamin D deficiency occurs
C treatment with folic acid produces complete recovery
D treatment with tetracycline is effective
E a clinical response to treatment commonly takes up to 6 months to develop

22. In the diagnosis between Crohn's disease and ulcerative colitis, the following findings would favour ulcerative colitis:

A involvement of the rectum
B stricture formation
C presence of eosinophils in the cellular infiltrate seen on biopsy
D 'cobblestone' appearance in barium enema
E crypt abscesses in biopsy

23. A patient in hospital with a relapse of his ulcerative colitis develops increasing fever, malaise and abdominal distension, with continued profuse diarrhoea:

A treatment with loperamide will be beneficial
B a plain X-ray of the abdomen is essential
C systemic corticosteroid therapy is absolutely contra-indicated
D surgical consultation is desirable
E evidence of superadded bowel infection should be sought

24. In the pathogenesis of infective diarrhoea

A jejunal biopsy of patients infected with Shigella dysenteriae shows necrosis of villus tip cells
B bacteria-free supernatant from a culture of V. cholerae can cause diarrhoea
C Salmonella spp. typically cause diarrhoea through mucosal invasion of the lymphoid tissue of the ileum
D persistent symptoms may be due to infestation with Ascaris lumbricoides
E C. perfringens ß antitoxin immunotherapy is effective

25. In a patient suspected of having acute appendicitis

A the finding of a segment of acutely inflamed ileum is diagnostic of Crohn's disease
B an appendix mass is best treated conservatively
C antibiotics have no place in the treatment
D symptoms and signs are often misleading in the elderly
E an inflamed retrocolic appendix may mimic a urinary tract infection

26. Diverticulosis of the colon

50% >50 - Kumar/Clark p142

A is found in about one-third of UK residents over the age of 60
B is declining in incidence
C occurs most frequently in the transverse colon
D is a common cause of massive bleeding from the colon in elderly subjects
E is always associated with thickening of the circular and longitudinal muscles of the colon

27. In acute pancreatitis

A serum amylase levels are within normal limits in about one-fifth of the patients
B hypocalcaemia implies a poor prognosis
C treatment with insulin may be necessary
D treatment with azathioprine may be the cause
E progressing to a fatal outcome, pain is always present

28. A pancreatic pseudocyst

A develops in more than half the patients who suffer from acute pancreatitis
B may cause jaundice
C over the course of 1-2 years will resolve spontaneously in 90-95% of patients
D if drained surgically, will inevitably lead to the formation of fistula
E may cause ascites

29. Recognised presentations of carcinoma of the pancreas include

A thrombophlebitis migrans
B bleeding from oesophageal varices
C splenomegaly
D acute pancreatitis
E diabetes mellitus

30. In the dissolution treatment of gallstones

A calcified gallstones do not dissolve
B only cholesterol gallstones are suitable
C radiolucent gallstones are always suitable
D the treatment should not be given during pregnancy
E the process may take up to 2 years

31. In Gilbert's syndrome

A plasma bilirubin levels will double if calorie intake is restricted for 48-72 hours
B a normal liver biopsy is essential for the diagnosis
C administration of phenobarbitone will cause a rise in plasma bilirubin
D bilirubin is absent from the urine
E some 20-30% of patients will develop hepatic cirrhosis by the time they reach the age of 50

32. In acute hepatic encephalopathy

A the degree of mental disturbance is closely related to the blood ammonia level
B symptoms may be precipitated by diuresis
C the presence of flapping tremor (asterixis is diagnostic
D EEG changes may be helpful in diagnosis
E protein should be withdrawn completely from the diet

33. In the treatment of primary biliary cirrhosis, the following agents have been shown to be of value:

A cholestyramine
B vitamin D
C corticosteroids
D azathioprine
E penicillamine

34. In auto-immune chronic active hepatitis

A the onset is usually insidious
B hypersplenism often occurs
C the liver is usually enlarged
D the serum alkaline phosphatase is usually normal
E a firm histological diagnosis based on liver biopsy is essential before treatment is started

35. In primary hepatocellular carcinoma

A a plasma α-fetoprotein level over 1 g/ml is diagnostic
B surgical resection is possible in only about 10% of cases
C X-irradiation may be expected to give remissions of up to 2 years
D the effect of cytotoxic drugs should be monitored by changes in the plasma α-fetoprotein
E the prognosis is better in Africa than in Western Europe

36. In amoebic abscess of the liver

A less than half the patients have amoebic trophozoites or cysts in their stools
B the right lobe of the liver is the more commonly affected
C the indirect fluorescent antibody test is positive in over 90% of patients
D the drug of first choice is metronidazole
E aspiration of the abscess hastens healing

37. In cystic fibrosis

A symptoms of pancreatic involvement may antedate respiratory manifestations by many years
B death from liver disease in early childhood is uncommon
C there is an increased incidence of gall-stones
D treatment with pancreatic extract can be expected to abolish steatorrhoea in nearly every case
E administration of ranitidine may be helpful

SECTION 13: CARDIOVASCULAR DISORDERS

1. **The following rhythm disturbances may arise as a result of digoxin toxicity:**

   A ventricular extrasystole
   B supraventricular tachycardia
   C atrioventricular conduction block
   D sinus bradycardia
   E atrial fibrillation

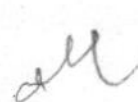

2. **The clinical features of pulmonary hypertension include**

   A haemoptysis
   B finger clubbing
   C cyanosis
   D parasternal heave
   E right ventricular failure

3. **Reversed splitting of the second heart sound may occur in**

   A pulmonary embolus
   B severe aortic stenosis
   C atrial septal defect
   D pulmonary stenosis
   E hypertrophic obstructive cardiomyopathy

4. **Complications of thiazide diuretics include**

   A gout
   B hypercalcaemia
   C photosensitive skin rashes
   D hyperglycaemia
   E hyperkalaemia

5. Pericarditis may be caused by

A thyrotoxicosis
B Dressler's syndrome
C tuberculosis
D left atrial myxoma
E pulmonary hypertension

6. In mitral valve prolapse

A there may be a typical chest pain
B ventricular ectopics are common
C there is a pansystolic murmur
D there is an increased risk of cerebral embolism
E prophylactic antibiotics should be given for dental procedures

7. The following statements are correct concerning Wolff-Parkinson-White syndrome:

A the syndrome is characterised by a short PR interval
B the QRS complex is narrowed
C there is a delta wave present
D in Type A Wolff-Parkinson-White syndrome there is a tall R wave in lead V 1
E both atrial fibrillation and A-V re-entrant tachycardia occur

8. Sick sinus syndrome

A is most common in middle age
B may cause tachycardias of supraventricular origin
C requiring cardiac pacing should be treated by ventricular rather than atrial pacing
D may be complicated by systemic embolism
E tachycardias often arise as an escape rhythm resulting from bradycardias

9. Infective endocarditis may cause the following extracardiac manifestations:

A glomerulonephritis
B splenomegaly
C confusional state
D meningo-encephalitis
E petechial haemorrhages

10. The following are major criteria for the diagnosis of rheumatic fever:

A carditis
B raised ESR
C polyarthritis
D first degree heart block
E fever

11. Aortic regurgitation may be due to

A ventricular septal defect
B ischaemic heart disease
C ankylosing spondylitis
D atrial septal defect
E thyrotoxicosis

12. Lignocaine

A may be effective in the treatment of supraventricular tachycardia
B is of proven value in the treatment of ventricular arrhythmias
C is a vasodilator
D may cause confusion
E may be given orally if long-term prophylaxis is required

13. The following are common features of amyloid heart disease:

A large voltage QRS complexes
B cardiomegaly
C no added sounds
D pulmonary venous congestion
E lack of response to digoxin

14. The following antibiotic regimens are effective in prophylaxis of infective endocarditis prior to dental extraction:

A amoxycillin 250 mg 6 hourly for one week prior to the extraction
B amoxycillin 3 g 1 hour before the extraction
C erythromycin 1.5 g orally 90 minutes before, then 500 mg orally six hours later
D amoxycillin 1 g one day before the extraction
E tetracycline 2 g one hour before the extraction

15. In pericardial tamponade

A sinus tachycardia is usually present
B arterial blood pressure falls in expiration
C there is evidence of pulmonary congestion on X-ray
D electrical alternans may be present
E the presence of a pericardial rub excludes a large effusion

16. A pansystolic murmur occurs in

A patent ductus arteriosus
B ventricular septal defect
C mixed mitral valve disease
D aortic regurgitation
E tricuspid regurgitation

17. Acute massive pulmonary embolism is commonly associated with the following clinical features:

A syncope
B a low arterial PO_2 and low arterial PCO_2
C a low arterial PO_2 and high arterial PCO_2
D left bundle branch block
E normal perfusion scan

18. The following are components of Fallot's Tetralogy:

A ventricular septal defect
B tricuspid atresia
C pulmonary stenosis
D left ventricular hypertrophy
E overriding aorta

19. The following are correct statements about the action of dopamine:

A low doses increase renal blood flow
B high doses cause bradycardia
C it increases myocardial O_2 demand
D it increases myocardial contractility
E it is ineffective in the treatment of chronic cardiac failure

20. The following are correct statements about atrial myxomas:

A they are always benign
B surgery carries a high risk
C they may present with signs identical to mitral stenosis
D they may present as pyrexia of unknown origin
E a 'tumour plop' may be audible in systole

21. In distinguishing between ventricular tachycardia and supraventricular tachycardia with aberrant conduction

A if there is evidence of independent atrial activity a tachycardia arising above the AV node can be excluded
B in patients with coronary artery disease a tachycardia with broad complexes is almost certain to arise from the ventricles
C if the configuration of an extrasystolic ventricular beat is similar to that during tachycardia, a common origin is probable
D supraventricular tachycardia is perfectly regular, whereas ventricular tachycardia is slightly irregular
E major haemodynamic disturbance occurs only with supraventricular tachycardia

22. The following factors increase the risk of ischaemic heart disease:

A hard water
B diabetes
C smoking
D low levels of LDL or total cholesterol
E moderate alcohol consumption

23. For amiodarone therapy the following statements are true:

A it is effective in treatment of supraventricular tachycardias
B it is effective in treatment of ventricular tachycardias
C its maximum therapeutic effect is seen in 48 hrs
D potentiation of warfarin occurs
E it has negative inotropic effect

24. The following are correct statements about hypertrophic cardiomyopathy (HOCM):

A it is inherited by an autosomal recessive gene
B the condition is characterised by a rapidly rising pulse
C typically it is associated with a pressure gradient between the body and outflow tract of the left ventricle
D arrhythmias should be sought and treated in every patient
E propranolol is contra-indicated

25. The following are correct statements concerning ventricular extrasystoles:

A they are more likely to represent coronary artery disease if they are unifocal
B they are more likely to be due to coronary artery disease if they occur on exercise
C the beneficial effect of anti-arrhythmic therapy for chronic ventricular extrasystoles is established
D the frequency of ventricular extrasystoles is related to prognosis in patients with coronary artery disease
E when they are associated with bradycardia, abolition of extrasystoles can be achieved by increasing the heart rate

26. The physical findings of an atrial septal defect include

A reversed splitting of the second heart sound
B wide fixed splitting of the second heart sound
C systolic murmur over pulmonary trunk, loudest in expiration
D pulmonary systolic click
E atrial fibrillation

27. In Beri-Beri heart disease

A thiamine therapy is curative
B venous pressure is raised
C pulse is of low volume
D there may be pulmonary oedema
E there may be a history of severe dietary deprivation

28. Cardiovascular syphilis

A causes calcification in the ascending aorta
B may cause coronary ostial stenosis
C when treated may be complicated by Herxheimer reaction
D may be accompanied by central nervous system involvement
E should be treated by a single dose of procaine penicillin

29. Dominant R wave in lead V1 of the ECG may be seen in

A pulmonary hypertension
B atrial septal defect
C left bundle branch block
D antero-septal myocardial infarction
E right bundle branch block

30. Easily preventable deaths due to hypertension may be due to

A cerebral haemorrhage
B dissecting aneurysm
C coronary artery disease
D myocardial infarction
E angina pectoris

31. Endocrine causes of hypertension include

A Cushing's syndrome
B Addison's disease
C Conn's syndrome
D Zollinger-Ellison syndrome
E phaeochromocytoma

32. The following drugs, widely used in the treatment of hypertension, act via the CNS:

A guanethidine
B captopril
C piretanide
D methyldopa
E clonidine

33. In the treatment of hypertension beta blockers

A are safe to use in all asthmatics
B lower morbidity following acute myocardial infarction
C have special advantages in bronchitis
D are the treatment of choice in women
E lower plasma renin in low doses

34. The following features suggest the need for further investigation in hypertension:

A abnormalities in plasma urea
B abnormalities in plasma potassium
C proteinuria
D glycosuria
E age of patient below 30 years

35. In predicting the surgical outcome in the treatment of renal vascular disease

A rapid sequence urography is of value
B isotope renography is of value
C divided renal function tests are of value
D captopril is of use
E determination of renal vein plasma renin may give false negative results

36. In a hypertensive patient, the following symptoms should arouse a suspicion of primary aldosteronism:

A muscular weakness
B thirst
C paraesthesiae
D oliguria
E tetany

37. Common symptoms (affecting 25% or more of patients) of phaeochromocytoma include

A headache
B palpitations
C sweating
D fear
E severe weight loss

38. Conditions producing symptoms suggestive of phaeochromocytoma include

A cerebral tumours
B hyperventilation
C hypothyroidism
D recurrent hypoglycaemia
E recurrent episodes of angina

39. Raynaud's disease (primary Raynaud's syndrome)

A occurs in males more often than in females
B commonly causes severe trophic changes in the extremities
C is commoner in the upper than in the lower limbs
D is usually symmetrical
E is not accompanied by organic arterial obstruction

40. In conventional cuff measurement of blood pressure

A the subject should always be supine
B the cuff should be about half the arm circumference
C a cuff width of 5 cm is suitable for a new born infant
D the cuff should be at the level of the heart
E there is a tendency to read above the true reading

41. First line investigation in hypertension is

A testing urine for protein or blood
B testing the pH of urine
C estimation of creatinine and electrolytes
D a chest X-ray
E recording of ECG

42. Calcium-blocking agents of use in treatment of hypertension include

A prazosin
B verapamil
C captopril
D nifedipine
E lidoflazine

43. Of value in the treatment of occlusive arterial disease

A are vasodilator drugs
B are anticoagulants
C is chemical sympathectomy
D is operative sympathectomy
E is reconstructive arterial surgery

44. The specific appearances of the fundus of the eye in hypertension include

A irregularity of the calibre of the arterioles
B 'cotton wool' spots
C increased light reflex (copper wire appearance)
D flame shaped haemorrhages
E arteriovenous nipping

SECTION 14: INTENSIVE CARE

1. Venous pressure increases in

A acute pulmonary embolus
B opiate intoxication
C obstructive airways disease
D medullary lesions
E diabetic ketoacidosis

2. Ventilation with positive end-expiratory pressure is contraindicated in

A low cardiac output states
B asthma
C pneumonia
D pulmonary oedema
E obstructive airways disease

SECTION 15: RESPIRATORY DISEASES

1. A large round mass in a chest X-ray might be due to

A hydatid cyst
B carcinoma
C extrinsic allergic alveolitis
D bronchogenic cyst
E Macleod's syndrome

2. Functional residual capacity will be increased in

A adult respiratory distress syndrome
B age
C asbestosis
D intra pulmonary airway disease
E ventilation with positive end-expiratory pressure

3. The effects of inhalation of silica on the lung include

A damage to type 2 pneumocytes
B decrease in synthesis of prostaglandins
C increased fibrosis
D increased adsorption of proteins
E granuloma formation

4. Clubbing is commonly found in

A silicosis
B talc pneumoconiosis
C cryptogenic fibrosing alveolitis
D uncomplicated bronchitis
E carcinoma of the lung

5. Corticosteroids are helpful in

A berylliosis
B cryptogenic eosinophilic pneumonia
C pulmonary alveolar proteinosis
D idiopathic pulmonary haemosiderosis
E allergic broncho-pulmonary aspergillosis

6. Effects of cigarette smoking on lung tissue and host defences include

A decrease in surface tension in acini
B increase in α antitrypsin
C increased risk of intrabronchial adenomas
D decrease in the number of alveolar macrophages
E destruction of alveolar walls

7. Pre-terminal bronchial epithelium contains the following cells:

A Clara cells
B goblet cells
C ciliated cells
D type I pneumocytes
E Feyrter cells

8. The following are acceptable as normal results:

A PO_2 100 mm Hg
B V/Q ratio: 1.0
C resting tidal ventilation 5 l/min
D FEV_1: 60% of vital capacity
E physiological dead space: 50% of tidal volume

9. Pleural fibrosis can be caused by

A empyema
B methysergide
C Goodpasture's syndrome
D hydatid disease of lung
E histoplasmosis

10. The following are correct statements concerning bronchial tumours:

A epidermoid (squamous) carcinoma is the most rapidly growing of all
B adenocarcinoma has the least association with smoking
C oat cell carcinoma can increase the release of ADH
D recurrent laryngeal nerve involvement is a contraindication for surgery
E hypertrophic pulmonary osteoarthropathy is uncommon in adenocarcinoma

11. Characteristic changes in emphysema include

A loss of elastic recoil of the lung
B decrease in total lung capacity
C increase in the transfer factor for carbon monoxide
D increase in residual volume
E air trapping

12. Pneumothorax

A is characterised by a negative Hamman's sign in an L.sided pneumothorax
B is common in Staphylococcus aureus pneumonia
C should always be treated with tube and drainage
D simplex is more common in young men
E almost never recurs after pleurectomy

13. Causes of unilateral hypertransradiancy include

A Macleod's syndrome
B an absent pectoral muscle
C acute alveolitis
D acute chickenpox pneumonia
E congenital absence of a pulmonary artery

14. Extrinsic allergic alveolitis may cause

A an increase in serum levels of IgG and IgM
B low ESR
C type I respiratory failure
D increase in blood eosinophil count
E diffuse fibrosis of the lung

15. Treatment for chronic respiratory failure due to chronic bronchitis should include

A controlled oxygen therapy
B digoxin
C diuretics
D long-term administration of carbonic anhydrase inhibitors
E corticosteroids

16. The following are correct statements concerning pleural effusions:

A in SLE, pleural effusion is nearly always unilateral
B practolol can cause pleural effusions
C tuberculous effusion has a low adenosine deaminase activity
D viral pneumonia is commonly accompanied by pleural effusions
E a right sided pleural effusion may occur in amoebiasis

17. The following are correct statements:

A pneumoconiosis is not associated with an increased risk of lung cancer
B calcification is a regular feature of coal worker's pneumoconiosis
C fibrosis in the asbetotic lung is predominantly in the upper zone
D the Kveim test is negative in berylliosis
E the upper permitted limit in the UK for respirable silica is 0.1 mg/cubic metre

18. Broncho-constriction in asthmatics may be caused by

A Aspergillus fumigatus
B ipratropium bromide
C prostaglandin F_2 alpha ($PGF_2\alpha$)
D prostaglandin E_2 (PGE_2)
E Dermatophagoides pteronyssimus

19. The following are correct statements:

A scoliosis is commoner in boys than in girls
B ankylosing spondylitis commonly presents with dyspnoea
C ankylosing spondylitis may be associated with pulmonary fibrosis
D pectus excavatum usually leads to respiratory failure
E in phrenic nerve paralysis the FEV_1 is usually normal

20. The following statements are helpful in making a diagnosis:

A when the PO_2 is less than 8 kPa and PCO_2 greater than 6.5 kPa respiratory failure is present
B the arterial-alveolar oxygen gradient is decreased in the adult respiratory distress syndrome
C diabetes insipidus is a manifestation of histiocytosis
D the circulating complement level is reduced in fibrosing alveolitis
E a bronchial carcinoid usually presents with a classical carcinoid syndrome

SECTION 16: RHEUMATOLOGY & CONNECTIVE TISSUE

1. Rheumatoid arthritis

A causes destruction of articular cartilage
B is frequently associated with the HLA antigen DR4
C is equally common in males and females
D is characterised by the presence of nodules
E can involve any synovial joint in the body

2. In rheumatoid arthritis

A ulnar nerve paralysis is due to entrapment of the ulnar nerve at the wrist
B general anaesthesia should be preceded by X-ray of the neck
C vasculitis occurs more often in patients with severe forms of the disease
D interstitial fibrosis of the lungs is the commonest form of pulmonary involvement
E pericarditis is common

3. The following are correct statements:

A in RA, anaemia is common and correlates with disease activity
B the anaemia of RA usually responds to treatment with iron and folate
C thrombocytopenia is common in untreated RA
D systemic lupus may first present as a haemolytic anaemia or as idiopathic thrombocytopenia
E thrombocytopenia is frequently seen in progressive systemic sclerosis

4. In occular involvement in the connective tissue diseases

A Sjogren's syndrome can occur in RA and SLE
B Sjogren's syndrome is associated particularly with the milder forms of RA
C scleromalacia perforans occurs more frequently in RA than Sjogren's syndrome
D acute anterior uveitis is often associated with ankylosing spondylitis
E uveitis is one of the usual presenting features of Reiter's disease

5. In ankylosing spondylitis

A there is at least 90% association with the tissue type HLA B27
B the inflammatory lesions start in the synovium
C the first symptom is always low back pain
D early morning stiffness is a marked feature
E the characteristic radiological changes of sacroiliac ankylosis always appear early

6. The following are correct statements about the sero-negative spond-arthritides:

A ulcerative colitis is frequently associated with polyarthritis
B ulcerative colitis and Crohn's disease may be associated with ankylosing spondylitis
C ankylosing spondylitis may be followed by inflammatory bowel disease
D keratoderma blennorrhagica is the characteristic skin lesion of Reiter's disease
E in psoriatic arthritis, skin lesions always precede the onset of arthritis

7. Systemic lupus erythematosus

A is commoner in Caucasian than in black women
B usually causes lymphopenia
C is always accompanied by immune complex deposition in the kidneys poor prognosis
D is rarely associated with central nervous system involvement
E should always be treated with corticosteroids

8. The following are correct statements:

A in polymyositis the presenting feature is usually progressive weakness in proximal muscles
B electromyography is usually diagnostic in polymyositis
C calcinosis is a frequent feature of adult dermatomyositis
D Raynaud's phenomenon is usually a presenting feature in scleroderma
E so far there is no proven curative treatment for scleroderma

SECTION 17: DISORDERS OF THE SKELETON

1. The following factors tend to cause proportionate rather than disproportionate (short-limbed) short stature:

A hypothyroidism
B Turner's syndrome
C hypophosphataemic rickets
D coeliac disease
E hypophosphatasia

2. The following are correct statements about osteoporosis:

A idiopathic juvenile osteoporosis is usually self-limiting
B osteoporosis due to Cushing's syndrome tends to spare the vertebrae
C the diagnosis should always be confirmed by bone biopsy
D in the treatment of established osteoporosis, oral calcium (1200 mg/day) is without serious side-effects
E hypercalciuria is sometimes found

3. In osteomalacia

A occurring in black immigrants, the primary cause is skin pigmentation
B the bones are always less dense than normal on X-ray
C due to hypophosphataemic vitamin D-resistant rickets, the best treatment is large oral doses of phosphate
D the plasma alkaline phosphatase may be normal
E the radiological hallmark of active disease is the Looser zone

4. In the clinical diagnosis between Marfan's syndrome and homocystinuria, the following findings would favour the latter

A sideways dislocation of the lens
B aortic incompetence
C mental retardation
D mitral valve prolapse
E osteoporosis

5. Recognised findings in polyostotic fibrous dysplasia (Albright's syndrome) include

A increased incidence in females compared with males
B sexual precocity
C dominant inheritance
D raised plasma phosphate
E raised plasma alkaline phosphatase

6. Radiographs in the following conditions may show bone sclerosis

A polymyalgia rheumatica
B alkaptonuria
C prolonged parenteral nutrition
D fluorosis
E osteopetrosis

SECTION 18: NEPHROLOGY

1. In testing urine with a dip-stick, it should be borne in mind that

A the protein detector is insensitive to Bence Jones protein
B the blood detector is insensitive to myoglobin
C the glucose detector is sensitive to any reducing sugar
D the pH detector may draw attention to the possibility that a positive protein result may be erroneous
E the nitrite detector tends to give false-positive results for urinary infection

2. The finding of pyuria with a negative urine culture could be explained on the basis of

A very dilute alkaline urine left at room temperature
B renal tuberculosis
C calculus in the bladder
D polycystic disease of the kidneys
E acute glomerulonephritis

3. Glomerular filtration rate

A exhibits a circadian rhythm
B is strictly proportional to the reciprocal of the plasma creatinine
C requires the collection of timed urine samples for its measurement
D doubles over the first two weeks of life
E declines during the last month of pregnancy

4. The following results are consistent with normal renal function in adults:

A protein excretion: 250 mg in 24 hours
B maximum urine concentration after 40 μg desmopressin intranasally: 750 mosmol/kg
C lowest pH of urine after ammonium chloride 100 mg/kg: 5.6
D plasma creatinine 120: μmol/l
E phosphate threshold: 1.0 mmol/l

5. A woman of 50 is referred by her general practitioner with a provisional diagnosis of diabetes insipidus. You would think that psychogenic polydipsia was more likely if you found

A a history of abrupt onset
B a plasma osmolality of 265 mosmol/kg
C a urine osmolality after dehydration (loss of 5% body weight) of 700 mosmol/kg
D failure of urine osmolality to rise after ADH injection
E absence of nocturnal polyuria

6. Idiopathic oedema of women

A is a manifestation of pre-menstrual tension
B always involves oedema of the ankles
C does not occur after the menopause
D may be precipitated by prolonged standing
E is best treated by diuretics in generous doses

7. Recognised causes of hypokalaemia include

A primary aldosteronism
B treatment with captopril
C liquorice addiction
D renal tubular acidosis
E digitalis intoxication

8. In acute glomerulonephritis in children

A the prognosis is good
B if a nephrotic syndrome develops it tends to persist
C crescent formation may be seen
D steroids are effective in arresting the progress of the disease
E proteinuria is usually less than 5 g/24 h

9. Minimal-change nephropathy

A is the commonest cause of the nephrotic syndrome in childhood
B does not relapse after remission
C produces highly selective proteinuria
D does not cause depression of the serum complement level
E must always be confirmed by renal biopsy

10. Renal involvement in Henoch-Schonlein purpura

A may cause macroscopic haematuria
B is rare in adults
C becomes arrested when the attacks of purpura cease
D causes changes in the renal biopsy specimen indistinguishable from those of IgA disease (Berger's disease)
E has been shown to be an immune response to antigens of Group A haemolytic streptococci

11. In renal amyloidosis

A the blood pressure is usually normal at presentation
B evidence of amyloidosis can always be obtained from rectal and gum biopsy if both tissues are sampled
C recurrence in a transplanted kidney is infrequent
D steroids and immunosuppressive drugs are ineffective
E proteinuria is usually poorly selective

12. Postural proteinuria in a child or young adult

A is usually highly selective
B is no longer thought to be benign
C accompanied by haematuria carries the same prognosis as isolated postural proteinuria
D may persist for several decades
E does not justify further investigation

13. In the management of the nephrotic syndrome

A patients with gross oedema under the age of 17 should be given prophylactic penicillin
B cellulitis is a medical emergency
C clofibrate should be given to all patients with hyperlipidaemia
D prophylactic subcutaneous heparin is advisable for patients in hospital
E oliguria with concentrated urine should be treated with protein replacement before diuretics are given

14. In the urethral syndrome in women

A pyuria does not occur
B urine culture is sterile
C the symptoms may be precipitated by sexual intercourse
D nocturnal frequency is a cardinal complaint
E energetic therapy with antibiotics offers the best prospect of relief

15. The following are correct statements about stone formation in the urinary tract:

A the commonest stones are those composed of magnesium ammonium phosphate
B in populations living at, or near, subsistence level, bladder stones in children are common
C in patients with recurrent stones, the rate of stone formation is higher in the winter than in the summer
D normal urine is supersaturated with respect to the ions that compose stones containing calcium and magnesium
E patients who have recurrent calcium-containing stones should maintain a water diuresis

16. In the management of idiopathic hypercalciuria

A treatment is not required unless it is associated with urolithiasis
B the patient should be advised to limit his or her intake of tea
C thiazide diuretics will reduce urinary calcium excretion
D administration of allopurinol is advisable in the majority of cases
E cellulose phosphate may cause obstinate constipation

17. Procedures effective in the emergency treatment of severe hypercalcaemic nephropathy

A infusion of isotonic sodium chloride
B administration of bendrofluazide
C oral administration of orthophosphate
D administration of mithramycin
E infusion of sodium sulphate

18. In the diagnosis of urinary tract obstruction

A satisfactory excretion urography cannot be performed if the blood urea is over 100 mg/dl
B false-positive results indicating hydronephrosis make ultrasound unacceptable as a screening procedure
C delay in the excretory phase of the renogram is not diagnostic of obstruction
D the late nephrogram is denser on the affected side if the obstruction is recent
E rectal palpation of the prostate is a reliable guide to the degree of obstruction caused by it

19. Administration of the following drugs in appropriate dosage carries a risk of renal damage:

A co-trimoxazole
B kanamycin
C cephalexin
D amphotericin
E methicillin

20. In analgesic nephropathy

A urinary sodium excretion is often very low
B women are more often affected than men
C proteinuria is usually slight
D persistent microscopic haematuria is probably due to papillary necrosis
E the best way of establishing the diagnosis is through renal biopsy

21. Special care with dosage is necessary when a patient with severe renal failure needs to be treated with

A amoxycillin
B erythromycin
C ibuprofen
D flucytosine
E propranolol

22. A man of 25 is admitted following a severe road accident in which he sustained multiple injuries. Forty-eight hours after admission, and following blood and fluid replacement thought on clinical grounds to be adequate, his urine flow is 0.4 ml/min. Your suspicion that he had developed acute tubular necrosis would be strengthened if you found

A urine osmolality 350 mosm/kg
B urine sodium 20 mmol/l
C urine/plasma urea ratio 3.5
D renal failure index 10.0
E fractional excretion of sodium 0.4%

23. In a patient with chronic renal failure, the following features would make renal transplantation inadvisable:

A generalised bronchiectasis
B adult polycystic kidney disease
C oxalosis
D chronic pyelonephritis
E patient aged 60

24. For a patient who has had a successful renal transplant the following are true:

A if immunosuppressive therapy is interrupted, even briefly, the graft may be lost
B an increased incidence of malignant disease must be expected
C if the patient develops hypertension, orthodox drug therapy will probably be ineffective
D the clinical manifestations of sepsis may be masked
E a GFR of 30-40 ml/min may be expected

25. In adult polycystic disease of the kidney

A inheritance is autosomal dominant
B hepatic cysts occur in about one-third of the patients
C the best technique for early recognition of cysts in a suspected case is ultrasound
D there is a substantially increased risk of death from intracranial haemorrhage
E percutaneous cyst puncture can substantially delay the onset of terminal renal failure

SECTION 19: DISORDERS OF THE BLOOD

1. The erythrocyte sedimentation rate

A is increased in pregnancy
B decreases with increasing age
C is raised in polycythaemia
D can be corrected accurately for changes in haemoglobin level
E is significantly affected by small departures from the vertical of the sedimentation tube

2. Red blood cells

A have a transverse diameter smaller than that of any capillary
B utilise ATP as an energy source
C continuously pump sodium out of their interior
D in adults normally contain 27-32 micrograms of haemoglobin each
E carry out glycolysis by means of the tricarboxylic acid cycle

3. Erythropoietin

A is a glycoprotein
B has been isolated in pure form
C is produced mainly by the kidney
D can be measured by radioimmunoassay
E is produced in increased amounts in response to tissue hypoxia

4. Characteristic features of the anaemia of chronic disorders include

A normocytic red cells
B low plasma iron
C high TIBC
D increased iron in reticulo-endothelial cells
E increased plasma copper

5. Alimentary absorption of iron is increased by

A ingestion of alcohol
B ingestion of egg
C ingestion of orange juice
D reduction of iron stores
E administration of tetracycline

6. The following are correct statements about iron metabolism and deficiency:

A in healthy adults the serum ferritin concentration is directly related to the available storage iron
B the serum iron level is a sensitive index in screening for idiopathic haemochromatosis
C a transferrin saturation of less than 16% is diagnostic of iron deficiency
D the finding of target cells in the peripheral blood of a patient with microcytic anaemia indicates that simple iron deficiency is not the cause
E the most sensitive index of the early stages of depletion of iron stores is the absence of stainable iron in the bone marrow

7. In idiopathic haemochromatosis

A the pigment causing darkening of the skin is haemosiderin
B the heart is usually enlarged
C in males, heavy haemosiderin deposits in the testis are usual
D mortality from primary carcinoma of the liver is strikingly reduced by repeated venesection
E intravenous desferrioxamine is the treatment of choice

8. Humans may obtain vitamin B_{12} from

A vegetables
B synthesis by intestinal bacteria
C eggs
D yeast
E cooked meat

9. Characteristic findings in pernicious anaemia include

A circular macrocytes in the blood film
B hypersegmentation of neutrophils
C a total leucocyte count of less than $1.5 \times 10^9/l$
D elevation of serum lactic dehydrogenase
E absence of haptoglobins

10. In homozygous ß-thalassaemia

A symptoms are usually first seen at the age of 9-12 years
B the haemoglobin F level is always raised
C even with adequate transfusion gross splenomegaly will develop
D without transfusion there is marked retardation of growth
E white cell and platelet counts are reduced when associated with hypersplenism

11. In idiopathic acquired sideroblastic anaemia

A the MCV is often raised
B the majority of cases have splenic enlargement
C there is usually a marked leukopenia
D splenectomy is beneficial if thrombocytopenia develops
E serum iron and ferritin levels should be monitored

12. G6PD deficiency

A is uncommon in South-East Asia
B forms the basis of favism
C commonly causes neo-natal jaundice in affected babies
D produces characteristic morphological changes in the blood even in the absence of haemolysis
E may be difficult to diagnose during an acute haemolytic crisis

13. Characteristic features of paroxysmal nocturnal haemoglobinuria include

A abdominal pain
B splenomegaly
C venous thrombosis
D hyperactivity of bone marrow
E autosomal recessive inheritance

14. In polycythaemia vera it is usual to find

A normal arterial oxygen saturation
B reduced leucocyte alkaline phosphatase
C reduced serum vitamin B_{12} content
D megaloblastic erythropoiesis
E defective haemostasis

15. The following are correct statements about leucocytes:

A the function of monocytes is to synthesise antibodies
B a circulating neutrophil count below 1.5×10^9 per litre indicates neutropenia
C T-lymphocytes have a longer life-span than B-lymphocytes
D eosinophils are phagocytic
E the granules of basophils contain antibody

16. In acute lymphoblastic leukaemia

A a mediastinal mass suggests T-cell ALL
B widespread lymph node enlargement may occur
C in patients under the age of 15, girls are more often affected than boys
D stained blood films commonly show Auer rods
E B-cell ALL has the best prognosis

17. In the induction of remission in acute lymphoblastic leukaemia

A the drugs used for standard risk patients should be vincristine and prednisolone
B failure to respond within four weeks implies a much worse prognosis
C the commonest complication is marrow failure
D treatment with allopurinol should be started before chemotherapy
E in the examination before treatment, rectal examination should never be omitted

18. In the management of acute non-lymphoblastic leukaemia

A priority should be given to restoring the haemoglobin level to normal by transfusion
B there is a serious risk of infection during the induction of remission
C fresh salads should not be given to neutropenic patients
D prophylaxis against CNS involvement should always be given
E a patient who has survived for five years or more can probably be considered as cured

19. In chronic granulocytic leukaemia

A most cases have thrombocytopenia when first diagnosed
B over 95% of cases have the Philadelphia chromosome
C the transformed phase may sometimes last for one or two years
D successful treatment with busulphan causes the spleen to become smaller
E there is clear evidence that splenectomy prolongs life

20. Specific therapy is called for in chronic lymphocytic leukaemia

A the lymphocyte count in the peripheral blood rises above 100 x 10^9/l
B the Coombs' test is positive
C there is increasing lymph-node enlargement
D the lymphocytes are found to be predominantly B-cell in type
E there is evidence of marrow failure

21. In the treatment of chronic lymphocytic leukaemia

A failure to respond to chlorambucil suggests that the diagnosis is wrong
B chlorambucil should not be used initially in patients presenting with marrow failure
C administration of prednisolone in high doses is hazardous in the elderly immunosuppressed patient
D radiotherapy is ineffective
E cyclophosphamide is usually less well tolerated than chlorambucil

22. The following are essential components of the intrinsic coagulation system:

A pre-kallikrein
B high molecular weight kininogen
C factor VII
D tissue factor
E factor XI

23. The activated partial thromboplastin time test is useful for the detection of deficiency of

A factor XI
B pre-kallikrein
C high molecular weight kininogen
D factor VII
E factor XII

24. In classical haemophilia

A female carriers can only be identified through the family history
B bleeding into the central nervous system is the commonest cause of death
C major surgery may be undertaken provided the factor VIII level is raised to 30% of normal
D pain in joints is best treated with indomethacin
E the response to desmopressin cannot be used to produce a long-term rise in factor VIII level

25. In the management of disseminated intravascular coagulation

A due to septicaemia, control of the infection usually causes the bleeding to stop
B heparin should usually be given
C platelets should not be given
D the diagnosis should be clearly established before treating the DIC itself
E due to abruptio placentae the uterus should be emptied

26. Heparin

A is a polypeptide
B carries a strong negative charge
C requires the presence of a plasma co-factor for its activity
D can be found in extracellular lung sites
E in low doses offers valuable protection against incipient peripheral arterial disease

27. The action of warfarin is potentiated by

A metronidazole
B cimetidine
C alcohol
D rifampicin
E clofibrate

28. In myelosclerosis

A the hyperplastic process spares the megakaryocytes
B splenomegaly is mainly due to myeloid metaplasia
C about one-third of patients show patchy osteoporosis
D poikilocytosis in the peripheral blood is usual
E the most effective way of reducing the size of the spleen is by radiotherapy

29. In idiosyncratic acquired aplastic anaemia

A the peripheral blood nearly always contains a few abnormal cells
B severe haemorrhage is unusual as a presenting feature
C a neutrophil count of $0.3 \times 10^9/l$ indicates a grave prognosis
D if bone marrow transplantation is to be carried out, the sooner it is done the better
E corticosteroids in high dosage should be given

30. Treatment is advised for the various stages of Hodgkin's disease as follows:

A Stage IA: radiotherapy
B Stage IB: chemotherapy
C Stage IIA: radiotherapy
D Stage IIIB: chemotherapy
E Stage IVA: chemotherapy

31. The prognosis in Hodgkin's disease is worse if the

A patient has fever on presentation
B patient is elderly
C patient is female
D histology is that of nodular sclerosis
E patient has been treated previously for Hodgkin's disease

32. Burkitt's lymphoma

A ocurs only in Equatorial Africa
B usually shows intra-abdominal involvement
C is extremely sensitive to chemotherapy
D can occasionally be cured
E usually involves the spleen and lymph nodes

33. Following a transfusion of incompatible blood

A serum haptoglobin levels fall
B methaemalbumin is formed in the blood
C the excretion of haemoglobin by the kidney causes renal damage
D jaundice may occur
E the most important aim of therapy (after stopping the transfusion) is to maintain the urine output

SECTION 20: DISEASES OF THE SKIN

1. The following skin diseases display autosomal dominant inheritance:

A hereditary haemorrhagic telangiectasia
B tuberous sclerosis
C phenylketonuria
D xeroderma pigmentosum
E neurofibromatosis

2. There is an association between erythema nodosum and

A staphylococcal infection
B sarcoidosis
C Crohn's disease
D diabetes
E steroid therapy

3. Subepidermal blisters are found in

A erythema multiforme
B toxic epidermal necrolysis
C pemphigus
D phemphigoid
E diabetes mellitus

4. The following statements concerning drug-induced lupus erythematosus are correct:

A it is characterised by high titre of antinuclear antibody
B DNA binding is high
C it is commonly irreversible
D it may be caused by phenytoin
E it may be caused by isoniazid

5. In psoriasis

A there is a tenfold increase in the speed of epidermal proliferation
B the lesion-free skin in affected patients is normal
C lesions may develop in traumatised skin
D arthropathy occurs in 7% of patients
E the edges of a lesion are usually the least active

6. In the management of psoriasis

A steroid creams are completely safe
B dithranol therapy always produces staining, and this is a sign of effectiveness
C natural sunlight is helpful in 75% of cases
D there is no increased risk of skin cancer in patients receiving PUVA therapy
E systemic steroids should be avoided if possible

7. Generalised increased pigmentation may be seen in the following:

A acanthosis nigricans
B chronic liver disease
C vitiligo
D ectopic ACTH secretion
E haemochromatosis

8. Scarring alopecia may be caused by

A secondary syphilis
B lupus erythematosus
C lichen planus
D psoriasis
E cyclophosphamide

9. Onycholysis may be seen in

A thyroid disease
B trauma
C Addison's disease
D psoriasis
E iron deficiency

10. Recognised complications of erythroderma include

A high output cardiac failure
B hyperthermia
C hypothermia
D pre-renal renal failure
E hypo-albuminaemia

11. Lichen planus

A is common in children
B typically first appears in the axillae
C is commonly associated with severe itching
D may be a complication of anti-tuberculous therapy
E usually resolves without treatment

12. Pyoderma gangrenosum may occur in association with

A Crohn's disease of the colon
B leukaemia
C rheumatoid arthritis
D venous stasis
E Behcet's disease

13. The following may cause leg ulceration:

A temporal arteritis
B hyperthyroidism
C polycythaemia
D syringomyelia
E tuberculosis

14. The following skin diseases are associated with internal malignancy:

A erythema nodosum
B dermatomyositis
C pyoderma gangrenosum
D acanthosis nigricans
E acquired ichthyosis

15. Recognised skin manifestations of sarcoidosis include the following:

A erythema multiforme
B lupus vulgaris
C chronic granuloma of the nose
D skin plaques
E epithelioid granulomas in the dermis

16. The following are correct statements concerning steroids used topically:

A halogenation decreases topical activity
B thinning of epidermis may occur
C thinning of dermis may occur
D systemic side-effects commonly occur
E the rate of epidermal turnover is increased

SECTION 21: NEUROLOGY

1. A CSF sugar content of less than 2.2 mmol/l may be found in

A tuberculous meningitis
B sarcoidosis
C carcinomatous meningitis
D subarachnoid haemorrhage
E cysticercosis

2. The common causes of unilateral central scotoma include

A papillitis
B optic nerve glioma
C papilloedema due to raised intracranial pressure
D parasellar meningioma
E glaucoma

3. Bilateral sixth cranial nerve palsies may occur in

A tuberculous meningitis
B nasopharyngeal carcinoma
C the Guillain-Barré syndrome
D raised intracranial pressure
E motor neurone disease

4. Bilateral facial weakness is a feature of

A the Guillain-Barré syndrome
B myasthenia gravis
C pontine glioma
D multiple sclerosis
E sarcoidosis

5. A lesion of the deep branch of the radial nerve may give rise to

A loss of sensation over the anatomical snuff-box
B weakness of flexor indicis
C depressed finger jerks on the side of the lesion
D weakness of extensor carpi ulnaris
E difficulties in abducting the fingers

6. Tetanus infection may give rise to

A tachycardia
B laryngeal spasm
C bradycardia
D apnoeic spells
E diarrhoea

7. In patients with transient ischaemic attacks in the carotid artery territory the risk of stroke is known to be reduced by

A anticoagulation with warfarin
B control of hypertension
C administration of aspirin 300 mg daily
D dipyridamole therapy
E giving up cigarette smoking

8. A lesion of the sixth cervical root is commonly associated with

A sensory loss over the middle finger
B weakness of biceps and brachioradialis
C a depressed or absent triceps jerk
D prolapse of the C6/7 intervertebral disc
E weakness of finger extension

9. In patients with cerebral abscess

A examination of the CSF is a useful investigation
B anaerobic bacteria are often cultured from intracranial pus
C steroid therapy is contraindicated
D the mortality rate is over 30 per cent
E there may be a history of congenital heart disease

10. The following conditions are inherited as autosomal dominant traits:

A neurofibromatosis
B Friedreich's ataxia
C hereditary spastic paraplegia
D tuberous sclerosis
E Leber's optic atrophy

11. Cherry red spots may be seen at the macula in

A metachromatic leukodystrophy
B Tay-Sach's disease
C ataxia telangiectasia
D Niemann-Pick disease
E Gaucher's disease

12. Multiple sclerosis

A affects both sexes equally
B may present with hemiparesis
C is often associated with a CSF protein of greater than 1 g/l
D commonly gives rise to depressed or absent tendon reflexes
E often relapses during pregnancy

13. In patients with Parkinson's disease

A there is a higher than average incidence of cigarette smoking
B there is loss of pigmented neurones in the substantia nigra and locus coeruleus
C tremor is decreased at rest
D symptoms which are unilateral initially usually remain so
E there is a good response to L-dopa in over 90 per cent

14. Wilson's disease

A may present with psychosis
B is characterised by high serum copper levels
C often causes pseudobulbar palsy
D is usually first diagnosed in the fifth decade
E is associated with abnormal tendon reflexes and plantar responses

15. Chorea may be associated with

A use of the contraceptive pill
B acanthocytosis
C myxoedema
D systemic lupus erythematosus
E polycythaemia rubra vera

16. The following drugs may induce the extrapyramidal disease indicated:

A diazoxide - acute dystonia
B reserpine - Parkinsonism
C lithium carbonate - tardive dyskinesia
D neuroleptics - akathisia
E tetrabenazine - tremor

17. The neurological manifestations of sarcoidosis include

A elevated protein level in the CSF
B meningeal infiltration
C myopathy
D multiple polyneuropathy
E bilateral Bell's palsy

18. The neurological complications of chronic renal failure include

A myoclonus
B proximal myopathy
C Parkinsonism
D dementia
E Ekbom's syndrome

19. Epileptic seizures

A occur at some time during the life of 1 in 30 of the population
B rarely occur after uncomplicated head injury
C may be precipitated by lack of sleep
D do not preclude the patient from holding a driving licence if consciousness is not impaired
E can often be distinguished from syncope on the basis of an EEG recorded between attacks

20. Typical absence (petit mal) seizures

A may develop in adult life
B are often associated with myoclonic jerks
C may be provoked by hyperventilation
D are characterised by a 3 Hz spike and wave discharge on the EEG
E are best treated with phenytoin

21. The following are recognised disadvantages of phenytoin therapy:

A alopecia
B hyperactivity in childhood
C the drug has to be administered at least twice daily
D reduced bioavailability of oral contraceptives
E coarsening of the facies

22. Cysticercosis in man

A commonly presents with epilepsy
B may cause hydrocephalus
C produces an eosinophilic pleocytosis in the CSF
D should not be treated with steroids
E may cause intermittent episodes of meningoencephalitis

SECTION 22: DISEASES OF VOLUNTARY MUSCLE

1. In Duchenne muscular dystrophy

A the mutant gene is of X-linked dominant inheritance
B the ECG may show evidence of right ventricular hypertrophy
C average intelligence is normal
D all mothers of affected boys are gene carriers
E carriers can be detected with certainty on the basis of creatine kinase estimation

2. Dystrophia myotonica

A is of autosomal dominant inheritance
B is associated with cataracts
C may cause mental retardation
D virtually always presents with myotonia
E is associated with glucose intolerance

3. Myasthenia gravis

A is caused by antibodies to the acetylcholine receptor in the majority of cases
B never remits spontaneously
C should be treated by thymectomy in most young females
D causes depression of the tendon reflexes
E may be associated with hyperthyroidism

SECTION 23: DISORDERS OF THE EYE

1. The following are correct statements about the fundal appearance in retinal disease:

A cotton wool spots represent accumulation of lipid and lipoprotein in the retina
B Roth's spots are a sign of subacute bacterial endocarditis
C flame shaped haemorrhages lie between the posterior vitreous face and the retina
D drusen are a sign of senile macular degeneration
E new vessels leak fluoresein dye intensively

2. Central retinal vein occlusion is associated with

A chronic simple glaucoma
B hypertension
C diabetes mellitus
D temporal arteritis
E retinal emboli

3. The following are correct statements about diabetic retinopathy:

A maculopathy is the commonest cause of visual loss
B ischaemic maculopathy can be helped by photocoagulation
C cotton wool spots often precede retinal neovascularisation
D laser treatment reduces visual acuity
E diabetic retinopathy improves during pregnancy

4. The following are correct statements about uveitis:

A 10% of patients with acute anterior uveitis are HLA B27 positive
B treatment consists of topical miotics and steroids
C hypopyon is a common feature of Behcet's disease
D in posterior uveitis the arteries are involved rather than the veins
E treatment with topical steroids can induce secondary glaucoma

5. With regard to the optic disc

A retinal axons are myelinated
B ischaemic optic neuropathy is caused by infarction of the posterior ciliary arteries
C reduced visual acuity is an early sign of papilloedema
D colour vision is reduced in papillitis
E in papilloedema the haemorrhages are restricted to the vicinity of the disc

6. With regard to glaucoma

A acute closed angle glaucoma is commoner in myopes than hypermetropes
B halos can precede the onset of chronic glaucoma
C reduction in visual acuity is an early sign of chronic glaucoma
D the upper end of normal intra-ocular pressure is 30 mm Hg
E secondary glaucoma can follow a central retinal vein occlusion

7. The following are correct statements about cataracts:

A cataract is the commonest cause of blindness in the world
B cataract is a feature of dystrophia myotonica
C cataract can follow uveitis
D posterior subcapsular lens opacities produce the least effect on visual acuity
E the posterior subcapsular region is the earliest site of change in steroid induced cataract

SECTION 24: DISORDERS OF UNCERTAIN AETIOLOGY

1. In Behçet's syndrome

A there is a strong association with HLA-B 5
B there may be recurrent deep venous thrombosis
C the skin may be hyperactive to minor injury such as venepuncture
D corticosteroid therapy is of definite value
E the condition is characterised by an inflammatory reaction around large blood vessels

2. In tuberous sclerosis

A there may be associated hydrocephalus
B abnormal calcification may be seen on the skull X-ray
C hamartomas in the lungs may give rise to spontaneous pneumothorax
D subungual fibromas commonly occur
E pulmonary involvement does not affect the prognosis

3. In recurrent polyserositis (familial Mediterranean fever)

A inheritance is by autosomal dominant transmission
B symptoms commonly start before the age of 20 years
C most patients manifest an asymmetric non-destructive monoarthritis
D colchicine has been established as the only effective treatment
E a skin rash resembling erysipelas occurs in 80% of patients

4. The following statements are true of retroperitoneal fibrosis:

A there is no recognised association with malignancy
B surgery is almost always necessary
C steroids may be helpful
D the only useful laboratory finding is raised ESR
E the ureters are displaced medially on IVU

SECTION 25: PSYCHIATRY AND MEDICINE

1. Tricyclic antidepressants

A may not produce any therapeutic effect for up to 3 weeks after starting treatment
B when failing to produce a response after four weeks should be continued for at least another four weeks
C are epileptogenic in predisposed patients
D commonly cause decreased sweating
E may cause tachycardia

2. The following are correct statements about alcohol dependence:

A increased tolerance of alcohol indicates that the subject is unlikely to develop dependence
B the earliest withdrawal symptom is tremulousness
C a dependent drinker is fully aware of his inability to control his drinking
D amnesic fugues are not pathognomonic of the condition
E once established its usual course is inexorable advance

3. The following factors are associated with high suicidal risk:

A age under 40 years
B persistent insomnia
C previous psychiatric history
D alcoholism
E epilepsy complicated by mood disorder

4. The following statements are correct concerning drug treatment of depression:

A MAOIs are more effective than tricyclic antidepressants for treatment of severe depressive illness
B when treating depression it is always preferable to start with tricyclic
C the therapeutic effects of MAOIs appear after three to five days
D foods containing tyramine should not be taken in conjunction with MAOIs
E MAOIs may cause orthostatic hypotension

5. Following bereavement

A there is usually a period of nonreaction followed by full reaction
B perceptual misinterpretations (illusions) are common
C death rate amongst bereaved close relatives is substantially increased
D atypical grief occurs mostly (80-90% of cases) in men
E in atypical grief the stage of nonreaction is often prolonged

6. Korsakoff's psychosis

A is usually associated with pyridoxine deficiency in chronic alcoholism
B may occur in association with severe vomiting
C involves damage to the mamillary bodies
D causes depression of consciousness
E causes gross impairment of long-term memory

7. The following drugs may cause erectile impotence in males:

A indomethacin
B L-dopa
C thioridazine
D propranolol
E probanthine

SECTION 26: SPORTS MEDICINE

1. Stress fractures

A the commonest site is the tibia
B X-rays may appear normal
C can be diagnosed using a physiotherapist's ultrasound applicator
D usually require rest for 3-4 weeks in a plaster of Paris cast
E bone scintigraphy is the most accurate diagnostic test

2. Soft tissue injuries

A should be treated by soaking in a hot bath followed by elevation
B usually need absolute rest for 1 week
C recover faster if non-steroidal anti-inflammatory agents are administered for 3-5 days
D following knee injury the quadriceps muscle may shrink by 30-50 per cent
E the presence of a torn anterior cruciate ligament of the knee is unlikely without a large haemoarthrosis

3. Exercise electrocardiography (ECG)

A correlates well with coronary arteriography results in asymptomatic men
B asymptomatic men with abnormal exercise ECGs are 10-20 times more likely to develop coronary disease than the general population
C is an efficient way of identifying at-risk joggers
D should be recommended regularly for all middle-aged sportsmen
E the mortality is about 1 in 3000

4. The following statements about amenorrhoea are true:

A it is commoner among athletes than among non-exercising women
B the more exercise taken the longer the luteal phase of the menstrual cycle
C amenorrhoea in athletes is due to low body weight
D exercise-induced amenorrhoea is always associated with loss of ovulation
E exercise-induced amenorrhoea frequently impairs future fertility

5. Exercise may induce the following abnormalities:

A anaemia
B hypovolaemia
C hyperthermia
D hypothermia
E hyperglycaemia

6. The following statements are true:

A raised plasma levels of creatine kinase, myoglobin, aspartate transaminase, lactate dehydrogenase and tropomyosin after a marathon are almost always due to myocardial infarction
B exertional rhabdomyolysis can cause acute tubular necrosis
C deficiency of carnitine palmityl transferase causes recurring exercise-induced rhabdomyolysis
D in renal failure due to rhabdomyolysis the plasma calcium level is high and the plasma phosphate low
E forced alkaline diuresis facilitates myoglobin excretion

7. The following statements about carbohydrate metabolism are true:

A the liver usually stores more glycogen than muscle
B sugar or glucose consumption just before endurance exercise is to be recommended
C fluids containing high glucose concentrations stimulate gastric emptying and therefore absorption
D during the second half of a marathon the runner depends on fat rather than glycogen for fuel
E adrenaline inhibits insulin secretion

SECTION 27: MEDICINE IN OLD AGE

1. In elderly patients with uncomplicated hypothermia

A tendon reflexes are normal
B the ECG shows prominent J-waves
C the principal manifestation is slowing of cerebration
D intravenous steroids are of benefit
E intravenous glucose is rapidly utilised

2. In the elderly

A drug absorption is, in general, reduced
B the effect of warfarin on synthesis of clotting factors is decreased
C potassium supplements should always accompany thiazide diuretic therapy
D renal tubular secretion of penicillin is increased
E the cardiac effects of propranolol are reduced

SECTION 28: TERMINAL CARE

1. The following are correct statements concerning the use of analgesics for terminal pain:

A aspirin is probably the most useful drug in the treatment of mild pain
B oral opiates are poorly absorbed
C diamorphine is superior to morphine in the treatment of severe pain
D opiates should be given at regular intervals to maintain adequate analgesia
E the addition of a phenothiazine to an opiate mixture may result in oversedation

2. In the treatment of raised intracranial pressure headaches

A high dosage steroids are the primary treatment
B the head of the bed should be lowered
C opiate analgesics should be avoided
D diuretics are of no therapeutic value
E anti-emetics acting on the vomiting centre, such as hyoscine, are useful in treating associated nausea

ANSWERS AND REFERENCES

Brackets indicate the correct answers. Against each lettered item is given the section and page reference to the Oxford Textbook of Medicine. For example: 4.1 (A) 4.10 indicates that in our Section 4 question 1 the answer A is correct and a full explanation of this item can be found in the Oxford Textbook of Medicine on 4.10 i.e. Section 4 page 10.

SECTION 4: GENETICS

4.1	(A)	4.10	4.2	(A)	4.39	4.3	(A)	4.4
	(B)	4.10		B	4.39		B	4.4
	C	4.11		C	4.39		C	4.4
	(D)	4.30		(D)	4.39		(D)	4.34
	E	12.140		(E)	4.38		(E)	4.35/4.4
4.4	A	4.24	4.5	(A)	4.90	4.6	(A)	4.99
	(B)	4.24		(B)	4.90		B	4.101
	C	4.25		(C)	9.27		C	4.102
	(D)	4.24		(D)	4.90		(D)	4.104
	(E)	4.28		E	9.30		(E)	4.103
4.7	(A)	4.107	4.8	(A)	4.108	4.9	(A)	4.127
	(B)	4.107		B	4.108		(B)	4.127
	C	4.107		(C)	4.108		C	4.127
	D	4.107		D	4.108		(D)	4.127
	E	4.107		(E)	4.95		E	4.127
4.10	(A)	4.132	4.11	A	4.134			
	(B)	4.132		(B)	4.134			
	C	4.132		(C)	4.134			
	(D)	4.132		D	4.134			
	E	4.133		E	4.134			

SECTION 5: INFECTIONS

5.1	(A)	5.4	5.2	(A)	5.6	5.3	(A)	5.18
	B	5.4		B	5.6		B	5.18
	C	4.82/5.2		C	5.6		(C)	5.18
	(D)	5.5		(D)	5.6		(D)	5.18
	(E)	5.5		(E)	5.6		E	5.19

5.4	A	5.19	5.5	A	5.20	5.6	(A)	5.36
	B	5.20		(B)	5.20		(B)	5.36
	(C)	5.19		C	5.20		(C)	5.36
	D	5.20		D	5.20		D	5.36
	E	5.20		E	5.20		(E)	5.36
5.7	A	5.49	5.8	A	5.54	5.9	A	5.59
	(B)	5.51		(B)	5.54		B	5.61
	(C)	5.66		(C)	5.54		(C)	5.61
	(D)	5.67		(D)	5.55		(D)	5.63
	(E)	5.71		E	5.54		(E)	5.63
5.10	A	5.68	5.11	(A)	5.69	5.12	(A)	5.72
	(B)	5.68		B	5.69		(B)	5.72
	C	5.68		(C)	5.69		(C)	5.73
	(D)	5.68		(D)	5.70		D	5.74
	(E)	5.69		E	5.69		E	5.73
5.13	(A)	5.76	5.14	(A)	5.80	5.15	(A)	5.85
	(B)	5.76		(B)	5.80		B	5.86
	(C)	5.77		C	5.81		C	5.86
	(D)	5.77		(D)	5.83		(D)	5.86
	(E)	5.78		(E)	5.80/5.83		E	5.88
5.16	A	5.89	5.17	(A)	5.117	5.18	A	5.95/ 5.138
	B	5.89		(B)	5.117		(B)	5.99
	C	5.89		(C)	5.117		(C)	5.97
	(D)	5.92		D	5.118		(D)	5.95
	E	5.91		E	5.119		(E)	5.98
5.19	A	5.106	5.20	A	5.123	5.21	A	5.136
	(B)	5.106		(B)	5.123		B	5.137
	C	5.108		(C)	5.123		C	5.137
	(D)	5.109		D	5.123		(D)	5.137
	(E)	5.109		(E)	5.124		(E)	5.138
5.22	(A)	5.139	5.23	(A)	5.141	5.24	(A)	5.148
	(B)	5.139		B	5.142		(B)	5.148
	(C)	5.140		(C)	5.142		(C)	5.148
	D	5.140		(D)	5.144		(D)	5.148
	E	5.141		(E)	5.143		(E)	5.148
5.25	A	5.164	5.26	(A)	5.171	5.27	(A)	5.175
	B	5.164		B	5.171		B	5.175
	(C)	5.165		C	5.171		C	5.175
	(D)	5.166		D	5.171		(D)	5.175
	(E)	5.168		(E)	5.171		E	5.175

5.28	(A) 5.182	5.29	(A) 5.192	5.30	(A) 5.196
	(B) 5.182		(B) 5.194		(B) 5.196
	(C) 5.184		(C) 5.194		C 5.196
	D 5.184		(D) 5.194		(D) 5.197
	(E) 5.187		E 5.194		(E) 5.197
5.31	A 5.199	5.32	(A) 5.202	5.33	A 5.208
	B 5.199		B 5.202		(B) 5.209
	C 5.200		C 5.202		(C) 5.210
	D 5.200		(D) 5.205		(D) 5.210
	(E) 5.201		(E) 5.205		(E) 5.210
5.34	A 5.210	5.35	(A) 5.211	5.36	A 5.213
	(B) 5.210		(B) 5.211		(B) 5.213
	(C) 5.210		C 5.212		(C) 5.213
	(D) 5.211		(D) 5.212		D 5.214
	E 5.211		E 5.212		(E) 5.214
5.37	A 5.214	5.38	(A) 5.214	5.39	(A) 5.218
	(B) 5.214		(B) 5.215		(B) 5.218
	C 5.214		(C) 5.215		(C) 5.218
	(D) 5.214		D 5.216		D 5.220
	E 5.214		(E) 5.215		(E) 5.218
5.40	A 5.219	5.41	(A) 5.226	5.42	A 5.233
	B 5.221		(B) 5.230		(B) 5.231
	(C) 5.220		C 5.230		(C) 5.231
	(D) 5.220		(D) 5.230		D 5.231
	(E) 5.220		(E) 5.230		E 5.233
5.43	(A) 5.234	5.44	A 5.239	5.45	(A) 5.246
	(B) 5.234		(B) 5.239		(B) 5.247
	(C) 5.235		C 5.239		(C) 5.248
	(D) 5.235		D 5.241		D 5.250
	E 5.236		E 5.241		E 5.250
5.46	A 5.255	5.47	(A) 5.260	5.48	(A) 5.265
	B 5.255		B 5.260		(B) 5.266
	(C) 5.256		(C) 5.261		(C) 5.266
	(D) 5.257		D 5.261		(D) 5.266
	E 5.257/5.258		E 5.265		E 5.270
5.49	(A) 5.278	5.50	A 5.280	5.51	A 5.305
	(B) 5.278		B 5.282		B 5.305
	(C) 5.278		(C) 5.282		(C) 5.306
	D 5.278		D 5.283		(D) 5.306
	E 5.279		E 5.285		E 5.306

5.52	A	5.387	5.53	A	5.399	5.54	A	5.327
	B	5.387		B	5.399		(B)	5.329
	C	5.387		(C)	5.399		C	5.328
	(D)	5.387		(D)	5.400		(D)	5.329
	E	5.389		(E)	5.400		E	5.331
5.55	A	5.637	5.56	(A)	5.636	5.57	(A)	5.423
	B	5.637		(B)	5.407		B	5.403
	C	5.638		(C)	5.334		C	5.361
	(D)	5.638		(D)	5.404		(D)	5.362
	(E)	5.639		(E)	5.371		E	5.463
5.58	A	5.332	5.59	A	5.406	5.60	A	5.410
	B	5.332		(B)	5.406		B	5.411
	C	5.331		C	5.406		C	5.437/ 5.411
	(D)	5.331/5.332		D	5.406		(D)	5.411
	(E)	5.333		(E)	5.406		E	5.410
5.61	(A)	5.364	5.62	A	5.341	5.63	(A)	5.379
	(B)	5.364		(B)	5.341		(B)	5.380
	C	5.510		C	5.341		(C)	5.378
	(D)	5.343		D	5.374		(D)	5.377
	(E)	5.373/5.375		E	5.341		(E)	5.381
5.64	(A)	5.426	5.65	(A)	5.432	5.66	(A)	5.362
	(B)	5.426		B	5.351		(B)	5.362
	(C)	5.427		C	5.352		C	5.370
	D	5.428		D	5.360		D	5.506
	E	5.426		E	5.333		E	5.561
5.67	(A)	5.551	5.68	(A)	5.455	5.69	(A)	5.427
	B	5.552		B	5.450		B	5.427
	C	5.553		C	5.525		(C)	5.427
	(D)	5.558		(D)	5.502		D	5.427
	(E)	5.566		(E)	5.561		E	5.427
5.70	(A)	5.366	5.71	A	5.317/5.452	5.72	(A)	5.459
	B	5.366		(B)	5.452		(B)	5.455
	C	5.366		(C)	5.452		(C)	5.458
	(D)	5.366		D	5.454		D	5.473
	E	5.366		E	5.450		E	5.511

5.73	(A)	5.547	5.74	A	5.409	5.75	A	5.596/ 5.599
	(B)	5.546		(B)	5.387		(B)	5.597
	(C)	5.546		(C)	5.507		(C)	5.598
	D	5.551		D	5.209		D	5.598
	E	5.552		(E)	5.99		E	5.596

5.76	A	5.371/5.420	5.77	(A)	5.446
	(B)	5.370		B	5.337
	(C)	5.371		(C)	5.471
	D	5.420		D	5.473
	(E)	5.421		(E)	5.533

SECTION 6: CHEMICAL AND PHYSICAL INJURIES, CLIMATIC AND OCCUPATIONAL DISEASES

6.1	A	6.149	6.2	A	6.16	6.3	(A)	6.128
	(B)	6.14		B	6.149/6.158		B	6.124
	C	6.15		(C)	6.152		C	6.89
	(D)	6.11		D	6.46		(D)	6.42
	(E)	6.14		E	6.151		E	6.160

6.4	(A)	6.56/6.4	6.5	A	6.96	6.6	A	6.54
	B	6.22		(B)	6.107		B	6.42
	(C)	6.11/6.4		C	6.131		(C)	6.152
	D	6.10		(D)	6.101		D	6.51
	E	6.29		E	6.70		(E)	6.12/ 6.152

6.7	(A)	6.15	6.8	(A)	6.113	6.9	A	6.13
	B	6.30		B	6.114		(B)	6.154
	C	6.44		(C)	6.114		(C)	6.154
	(D)	6.14		D	6.114/5.499		D	6.47
	E	6.154/6.156		(E)	6.114		(E)	6.154

6.10	(A)	6.45	6.11	A	6.54	6.12	A	6.150
	B	6.45		(B)	6.47		(B)	6.157
	C	6.45		C	6.53		C	6.13
	(D)	6.46		D	6.43		(D)	6.157
	E	6.45		(E)	6.152		(E)	6.157

6.13	(A)	6.143
	B	6.155
	C	6.156
	(D)	6.143
	(E)	6.143

SECTION 7: CLINICAL PHARMACOLOGY

7.1	(A)	7.1	7.2	(A)	7.7
	B	7.1		B	7.7
	(C)	7.1		C	7.7
	(D)	7.1		D	7.7
	E	7.15		(E)	7.7

SECTION 8: NUTRITION

8.1	(A)	8.6	8.2	(A)	8.9	8.3	A	8.9
	(B)	8.6		B	8.9		(B)	8.9
	C	8.6		(C)	8.9		C	8.9
	D	8.8		(D)	8.9		(D)	8.9
	(E)	8.6		E	8.10		(E)	8.9
8.4	(A)	8.12	8.5	A	8.14	8.6	(A)	8.17
	(B)	8.12		(B)	8.14		(B)	8.17
	(C)	8.12		(C)	8.13		C	8.17
	(D)	8.12		(D)	8.14		(D)	8.17
	(E)	8.12		E	8.14		(E)	8.18
8.7	(A)	8.39	8.8	A	8.27	8.9	A	8.25
	(B)	8.39		B	8.27		(B)	8.25
	(C)	8.39		(C)	8.24		(C)	8.25
	D	8.42		(D)	8.24		(D)	8.25
	(E)	8.39		(E)	8.24		E	8.25
8.10	(A)	8.25	8.11	(A)	8.27	8.12	(A)	8.35
	(B)	8.25		(B)	8.27		(B)	8.35
	(C)	8.25		(C)	8.27		(C)	8.35
	D	8.25		D	8.27		D	8.35
	E	8.25		E	8.27		(E)	8.35
8.13	(A)	8.55	8.14	(A)	8.30			
	B	8.55		(B)	8.30			
	C	8.55		(C)	8.30			
	(D)	8.55		D	8.30			
	(E)	8.55		(E)	8.30			

SECTION 9: METABOLIC DISORDERS

Question	Answer	Reference
9.1	(A)	9.55
	B	9.56
	(C)	9.55
	(D)	9.55
	E	9.56
9.2	(A)	9.59
	(B)	9.59
	C	9.59
	(D)	9.59
	E	9.59
9.3	(A)	9.61
	(B)	9.61
	C	9.61
	D	9.61
	(E)	9.61
9.4	(A)	9.68
	B	9.68
	(C)	9.68
	D	9.68
	E	9.68
9.5	(A)	9.69
	B	9.69
	C	9.70
	(D)	9.69
	E	9.70
9.6	(A)	9.71
	(B)	9.70
	C	9.71
	(D)	9.72
	E	9.74
9.7	A	9.72
	(B)	9.72
	(C)	9.72
	D	9.72
	(E)	9.72
9.8	A	9.71
	(B)	9.71
	(C)	9.71
	D	9.71
	E	9.71
9.9	A	9.78
	(B)	9.78
	C	9.78
	(D)	9.78
	E	9.78
9.10	A	9.83
	(B)	9.83
	(C)	9.83
	D	9.83
	(E)	9.83
9.11	(A)	9.91
	(B)	9.91
	C	9.91
	D	9.91
	(E)	9.91
9.12	(A)	9.98
	(B)	9.98
	C	9.99
	D	9.97
	(E)	9.98
9.13	A	9.108
	(B)	9.108
	(C)	9.108
	(D)	9.108
	(E)	9.108
9.14	(A)	9.129
	B	9.129
	(C)	9.129
	(D)	9.129
	E	9.129
9.15	A	9.139
	(B)	9.142
	C	9.139
	(D)	9.142
	E	9.141
9.16	(A)	9.48
	B	9.48
	C	9.50
	D	9.50
	(E)	9.50
9.17	(A)	9.167
	(B)	9.167
	C	9.167
	(D)	9.167
	(E)	9.167

SECTION 10: ENDOCRINE DISORDERS

10.1	(A)	10.12	10.2	(A)	10.20	10.3	(A)	10.28
	(B)	10.12		B	10.20		(B)	10.28
	C	10.18		(C)	10.20		(C)	10.28
	(D)	10.12		(D)	10.20		(D)	10.28
	E	10.12		(E)	10.20		(E)	10.28
10.4	A	10.36	10.5	(A)	10.42	10.6	A	10.38
	B	10.36		B	10.42		(B)	10.39
	(C)	10.36		C	10.42		(C)	10.39
	(D)	10.36		(D)	10.42		D	10.38
	(E)	10.36		(E)	10.42		E	10.44
10.7	(A)	10.39	10.8	(A)	10.43	10.9	A	10.53
	B	10.39		(B)	10.43		(B)	10.54
	C	10.39		(C)	10.43		(C)	10.54
	D	10.39		D	10.43		(D)	10.54
	(E)	10.39		(E)	10.44		E	10.54
10.10	(A)	10.71	10.11	A	10.72	10.12	A	10.96
	(B)	10.71		B	10.72		(B)	10.90
	C	10.71		C	10.72		C	10.97
	(D)	10.71		(D)	10.73		D	10.97
	(E)	10.70		(E)	10.73		E	10.97
10.13	(A)	10.89	10.14	A	10.86/10.89	10.15	(A)	10.93
	(B)	10.89		(B)	10.87		(B)	10.93
	C	10.89		C	10.87		C	10.77
	(D)	10.89		(D)	10.87		(D)	10.93
	(E)	10.89		E	10.86		(E)	10.93

SECTION 11: REPRODUCTIVE MEDICINE

11.1	(A)	11.1	11.2	(A)	11.2	11.3	A	11.8
	(B)	11.1		B	11.2		(B)	11.8
	C	11.3		(C)	11.2		(C)	11.8
	(D)	11.1		(D)	11.2		D	11.8
	E	11.3		(E)	11.2		(E)	11.8
11.4	A	11.9	11.5	A	11.12	11.6	(A)	11.23
	(B)	11.9		(B)	11.12		(B)	11.23
	(C)	11.9		C	11.13		(C)	11.23
	D	11.9		D	11.13		(D)	11.23
	(E)	11.9		E	11.13		(E)	11.23

SECTION 12: GASTROENTEROLOGY

Question	Option	Reference
12.1	(A)	12.17
	(B)	12.17
	C	12.17
	D	12.17
	(E)	12.17
12.2	(A)	12.23
	B	12.23
	(C)	12.23
	D	12.23
	E	12.24
12.3	A	12.41
	(B)	12.41
	(C)	12.41
	(D)	12.41
	(E)	12.41
12.4	(A)	12.44
	B	12.45
	(C)	12.45
	D	12.146
	E	12.45
12.5	A	12.46
	B	12.46
	C	12.46
	(D)	12.46
	E	12.46
12.6	A	12.50
	B	12.50
	(C)	12.50
	(D)	12.50
	(E)	12.50
12.7	(A)	12.53
	(B)	12.53
	C	12.69
	(D)	12.64
	E	12.53
12.8	(A)	12.56
	B	12.56
	(C)	12.56
	D	12.57
	E	12.57
12.9	(A)	12.55
	B	12.55
	(C)	12.55
	D	12.55
	E	12.55
12.10	(A)	12.53
	(B)	12.53
	C	12.53
	(D)	12.53
	(E)	12.53
12.11	(A)	12.58
	B	12.59
	(C)	12.59
	(D)	12.59
	(E)	12.58
12.12	(A)	12.59
	(B)	12.59
	(C)	12.59
	(D)	12.60
	(E)	12.60/ 12.259
12.13	A	12.66
	(B)	12.66
	C	12.66
	(D)	12.66
	(E)	12.66
12.14	(A)	12.67
	(B)	12.67
	(C)	12.67
	D	12.67
	E	12.67
12.15	A	12.22
	(B)	12.22
	(C)	12.22
	D	12.21
	(E)	12.21
12.16	A	12.66
	(B)	12.66
	C	12.71
	(D)	12.71
	E	12.71
12.17	(A)	12.74
	(B)	12.73
	(C)	12.74
	D	12.74
	E	12.74
12.18	(A)	12.88
	B	12.88
	(C)	12.88
	(D)	12.88
	(E)	12.88
12.19	(A)	12.111
	B	12.100
	(C)	12.100
	(D)	12.100
	(E)	12.100
12.20	(A)	12.105
	B	12.105
	(C)	12.105
	D	12.106
	(E)	12.105
12.21	A	12.118
	(B)	12.118
	C	12.116
	(D)	12.116
	E	12.120

Question	Answer	Reference
12.22	(A)	12.124
	B	12.124
	(C)	12.124
	D	12.124
	(E)	12.124
12.23	A	12.129
	(B)	12.129
	C	12.130
	(D)	12.132
	(E)	12.129
12.24	A	12.166
	(B)	12.166
	(C)	12.166
	(D)	12.168
	E	12.170
12.25	A	12.180
	(B)	12.180
	C	12.180
	(D)	12.179
	(E)	12.179
12.26	(A)	12.135
	B	12.135
	C	12.135
	(D)	12.137
	E	12.135
12.27	(A)	12.186
	(B)	12.185
	(C)	12.187
	(D)	12.184
	E	12.184
12.28	(A)	12.184
	(B)	12.184
	C	12.184
	D	12.192
	(E)	12.184
12.29	(A)	12.193
	(B)	12.193
	(C)	12.193
	(D)	12.193
	(E)	12.193
12.30	(A)	12.201
	(B)	12.201
	C	12.201
	(D)	12.201
	(E)	12.201
12.31	(A)	12.209
	B	12.209
	C	12.209
	(D)	12.208
	E	12.209
12.32	A	12.235
	(B)	12.235
	C	12.235
	(D)	12.235
	(E)	12.235
12.33	(A)	12.234
	(B)	12.234
	C	12.234
	D	12.234
	(E)	12.234
12.34	(A)	12.223
	(B)	12.223
	C	12.223
	(D)	12.223
	E	12.223
12.35	A	12.256
	(B)	12.257
	C	12.257
	(D)	12.257
	E	12.257
12.36	(A)	12.261
	(B)	12.261
	(C)	12.261
	(D)	12.261
	E	12.261
12.37	(A)	12.195
	(B)	12.196
	(C)	12.195
	D	12.196
	(E)	12.196

SECTION 13: CARDIOVASCULAR DISORDERS

13.1	(A)	13.104	13.2	(A)	13.346	13.3	A	13.357
	(B)	13.104		B	13.346		(B)	13.294
	(C)	13.104		C	13.346		C	13.271
	(D)	13.104		(D)	13.346		D	13.265
	(E)	13.104		(E)	13.346		(E)	13.224
13.4	(A)	13.100	13.5	A	13.305	13.6	(A)	13.291
	(B)	13.100		(B)	13.305		(B)	13.291
	(C)	13.100		(C)	13.305		C	13.291
	(D)	13.100		D	13.306		(D)	13.291
	E	13.100		E	13.348		(E)	13.291
13.7	(A)	13.123	13.8	A	13.129	13.9	(A)	13.318
	B	13.123		(B)	13.129		(B)	13.318
	(C)	13.123		C	13.130		(C)	13.318
	(D)	13.124		(D)	13.130		(D)	13.318
	(E)	13.124		(E)	13.129		(E)	13.318
13.10	(A)	13.279	13.11	(A)	13.296	13.12	A	13.133
	B	13.279		B	13.296		(B)	13.133
	(C)	13.279		(C)	13.296		C	13.133
	D	13.279		D	13.296		(D)	13.133
	E	13.279		E	13.296		E	13.133
13.13	A	13.202	13.14	A	13.324	13.15	(A)	13.308
	B	13.201		(B)	13.324		B	13.308
	(C)	13.202		(C)	13.324		C	13.308
	(D)	13.203		D	13.324		(D)	13.308
	(E)	13.204		E	13.324		E	13.308
13.16	A	13.276	13.17	(A)	13.356	13.18	(A)	13.243
	(B)	13.275		(B)	13.356		B	13.243
	(C)	13.287		C	13.356		(C)	13.243
	D	13.296		D	13.356		D	13.243
	(E)	13.301		E	13.358		(E)	13.243
13.19	(A)	13.114	13.20	(A)	13.312	13.21	(A)	13.126
	B	13.114		B	13.313		(B)	13.126
	(C)	13.114		(C)	13.312		(C)	13.126
	(D)	13.114		(D)	13.313		D	13.126
	E	13.114		E	13.313		E	13.126

13.22
A 13.149
(B) 13.146
(C) 13.148
D 13.146
E 13.149

13.23
(A) 13.134
(B) 13.134
C 13.134
(D) 13.135
E 13.134

13.24
A 13.221
(B) 13.223
(C) 13.225
(D) 13.228
E 13.228

13.25
A 13.119
B 13.119
C 13.119
(D) 13.119
(E) 13.119

13.26
A 13.271
(B) 13.271
C 13.271
(D) 13.271
(E) 13.271

13.27
(A) 13.403
(B) 13.403
C 13.403
(D) 13.403
(E) 13.403

13.28
(A) 13.325
(B) 13.326
(C) 13.326
(D) 13.326
E 13.326

13.29
(A) 13.346
(B) 13.272
C 13.26
D 13.30
(E) 13.26

13.30
(A) 13.360
(B) 13.360
C 13.360
D 13.362
E 13.362

13.31
(A) 13.390
B 10.76
(C) 13.390
D 12.68
(E) 13.392

13.32
(A) 13.380
B 13.380
C 13.381
(D) 13.374
(E) 13.374

13.33
A 13.378
(B) 13.374
C 13.374
D 13.374
(E) 13.379

13.34
(A) 13.383
(B) 13.383
(C) 13.383
(D) 13.383
(E) 13.383

13.35
A 13.386
B 13.386
C 13.386
(D) 13.386
(E) 13.386

13.36
(A) 13.390
(B) 13.390
(C) 13.390
D 13.390
(E) 13.390

13.37
(A) 13.394
(B) 13.394
(C) 13.394
(D) 13.394
E 13.394

13.38
(A) 13.394
(B) 13.394
C 13.394
(D) 13.394
(E) 13.394

13.39
A 13.185
B 13.185
(C) 13.185
(D) 13.185
(E) 13.185

13.40
A 13.363
(B) 13.363
C 13.363
(D) 13.362
E 13.363

13.41
(A) 13.383
B 13.383
(C) 13.383
(D) 13.383
(E) 13.383

13.42
A 13.379
(B) 13.380
C 13.380
(D) 13.380
(E) 13.376

13.43
A 13.188
B 13.188
(C) 13.189
(D) 13.189
(E) 13.188

13.44
(A) 13.369
(B) 13.369
C 13.369
(D) 13.369
E 13.369

SECTION 14: INTENSIVE CARE

14.1	(A) 14.7	14.2	(A) 14.13
	B 14.2		(B) 14.13
	(C) 14.10		C 14.13
	D 14.3		D 14.13
	E 14.2		(E) 14.11

SECTION 15: RESPIRATORY DISEASES

15.1	(A) 15.18	15.2	A 15.164	15.3	(A) 15.112
	(B) 15.18		(B) 15.35		B 15.40
	C 15.122		C 15.114		(C) 15.112
	(D) 15.18		(D) 15.31		(D) 15.41
	E 15.66		(E) 15.165		E 15.42
15.4	A 15.113	15.5	(A) 15.116	15.6	(A) 15.44
	(B) 15.115		(B) 15.131		B 15.44
	(C) 15.124		C 15.139		C 15.156
	D 15.51		D 15.130		D 15.44
	(E) 15.149		(E) 15.81		(E) 15.44
15.7	(A) 15.5	15.8	(A) 15.28	15.9	(A) 15.104
	B 15.5		B 15.28		(B) 15.144
	(C) 15.5		(C) 15.25		C 15.129
	D 15.6		D 15.32		D 15.173
	(E) 15.4		E 15.34		(E) 15.172
15.10	A 15.146	15.11	(A) 15.85	15.12	A 15.54
	(B) 15.146		B 15.86		(B) 15.98
	(C) 15.146/15.148		C 15.86		C 15.55
	(D) 15.153		(D) 15.86		(D) 15.54
	E 15.149		(E) 15.86		(E) 15.55
15.13	(A) 15.66	15.14	A 15.121	15.15	(A) 15.169
	(B) 15.67		B 15.121		B 15.84
	C 15.67		(C) 15.122		(C) 15.169
	D 15.67		D 15.121		D 15.169
	(E) 15.67		(E) 15.120		E 15.84
15.16	A 15.126	15.17	(A) 15.111	15.18	(A) 15.81
	(B) 15.144		B 15.111		(B) 15.142
	C 15.57		C 15.114		(C) 15.79/ 15.142
	D 15.98		(D) 15.116		D 15.79
	(E) 15.172		(E) 15.113		(E) 15.79

15.19	A 15.58	15.20	(A) 15.167		
	B 15.60		B 15.164		
	(C) 15.60		(C) 15.135		
	D 15.61		D 15.124		
	E 15.63		E 15.146		

SECTION 16: RHEUMATOLOGY AND CONNECTIVE TISSUE DISORDERS

16.1	(A) 16.3	16.2	A 16.3	16.3	(A) 16.8
	(B) 16.1		(B) 16.6		B 16.8
	C 16.3		(C) 16.7		C 16.8
	(D) 16.2/16.7		D 16.7		(D) 16.25
	(E) 16.3		(E) 16.8		E 16.35

16.4	(A) 16.8	16.5	(A) 16.11	16.6	A 16.19
	B 16.9		B 16.12		(B) 16.19
	C 16.9		C 16.12		(C) 16.19
	(D) 16.13		(D) 16.12		(D) 16.17
	E 16.17		E 16.13		E 16.15

16.7	A 16.20	16.8	(A) 16.48
	(B) 16.26		(B) 16.49
	(C) 16.24		C 16.49
	D 16.23		(D) 16.35
	E 16.26		(E) 16.40

SECTION 17: DISORDERS OF THE SKELETON

17.1	(A) 17.6	17.2	(A) 17.13	17.3	A 17.17
	(B) 17.6		B 17.13		B 17.16
	C 17.6		C 17.11		C 17.18
	(D) 17.6		(D) 17.13		(D) 17.16
	E 17.6		(E) 17.11		(E) 17.16

17.4	A 17.28	17.5	(A) 17.33	17.6	A 16.52
	B 17.28		(B) 17.33		B 17.30
	(C) 17.28/17.30		C 17.33		C 17.36
	D 17.28		D 17.33		(D) 17.35
	(E) 17.28/17.30		(E) 17.33		(E) 17.31

SECTION 18: NEPHROLOGY

18.1
(A) 18.1
B 18.1
C 18.1
(D) 18.2
E 18.2

18.2
A 18.2
(B) 18.2
(C) 18.2
(D) 18.2
(E) 18.2

18.3
(A) 18.5
B 18.5
C 18.5
(D) 18.15
(E) 18.16

18.4
A 18.7
(B) 18.8
C 18.8
(D) 18.6
(E) 18.9

18.5
A 18.23
(B) 18.23
(C) 18.23
D 18.23
(E) 18.23

18.6
A 18.29
B 18.29
C 18.29
(D) 18.29
E 18.29

18.7
(A) 18.31
B 18.35
(C) 18.31
(D) 18.31
E 18.36

18.8
(A) 18.41
B 18.41
(C) 18.41
D 18.42
(E) 18.41

18.9
(A) 18.44
B 18.44
(C) 18.45
(D) 18.45
E 18.45

18.10
(A) 18.47
(B) 18.47
C 18.47
(D) 18.47
E 18.47

18.11
(A) 18.53
B 18.53
(C) 18.53
(D) 18.53
(E) 18.53

18.12
A 18.57
B 18.57
(C) 18.57
(D) 18.57
(E) 18.57

18.13
(A) 18.63
(B) 18.63
C 18.63
(D) 18.63
(E) 18.63

18.14
A 18.70
(B) 18.70
(C) 18.70
D 18.70
E 18.70

18.15
A 18.88
(B) 18.87
C 18.88
(D) 18.88
(E) 18.88

18.16
(A) 18.94
(B) 18.94
(C) 18.94
D 18.94
E 18.94

18.17
(A) 18.95
B 18.95
C 18.95
(D) 18.95
(E) 18.95

18.18
A 18.102
B 18.101
(C) 18.102
(D) 18.103
E 18.100

18.19
(A) 18.111
(B) 18.111
C 18.111
(D) 18.111
(E) 18.111

18.20
A 18.113
(B) 18.113
(C) 18.113
D 18.113
E 18.115

18.21
(A) 18.123
B 18.123
C 18.123
(D) 18.123
E 18.123

18.22
(A) 18.125
B 18.125
(C) 18.125
(D) 18.125
E 18.125

18.23
(A) 18.149
B 18.149
(C) 18.149
D 18.149
(E) 18.149

18.24
(A) 18.153
(B) 18.155
C 18.155
(D) 18.154
(E) 18.153

Question	Option	Reference
18.25	(A)	18.164
	(B)	18.164
	C	18.164
	(D)	18.164
	E	18.164

SECTION 19: DISORDERS OF THE BLOOD

Question	Option	Reference
19.1	(A)	19.6
	B	19.6
	C	19.6
	D	19.6
	(E)	19.6
19.2	A	19.64
	(B)	19.65
	(C)	19.64
	D	19.4
	E	19.65
19.3	(A)	19.64
	(B)	19.64
	(C)	19.64
	(D)	19.64
	(E)	19.64
19.4	(A)	19.92
	(B)	19.92
	C	19.92
	(D)	19.92
	(E)	19.92
19.5	(A)	19.88
	B	19.80
	(C)	19.80
	(D)	19.81
	E	19.81
19.6	(A)	19.83
	(B)	19.88
	C	19.84
	D	19.85
	E	19.86
19.7	A	19.87
	(B)	19.87
	C	19.87
	D	19.88
	E	19.88
19.8	A	19.94
	B	19.94
	(C)	19.94
	D	19.94
	(E)	19.94
19.9	A	19.102
	(B)	19.102
	C	19.102
	(D)	19.102
	(E)	19.102
19.10	A	19.112
	(B)	19.113
	C	19.113
	(D)	19.113
	(E)	19.113
19.11	(A)	19.132
	B	19.132
	C	19.132
	D	19.133
	(E)	19.132
19.12	A	19.140
	(B)	19.141
	(C)	19.141
	D	19.141
	(E)	19.141
19.13	(A)	19.55
	B	19.57
	(C)	19.55
	D	19.55
	E	19.54
19.14	(A)	19.38
	B	19.38
	C	19.38
	D	19.38
	(E)	19.37
19.15	A	19.161
	(B)	19.159
	(C)	19.161
	(D)	19.162
	E	19.162
19.16	(A)	19.18
	(B)	19.18
	C	19.16
	D	19.20
	E	19.23
19.17	(A)	19.23
	B	19.23
	C	19.23
	(D)	19.23
	E	19.19
19.18	A	19.26
	(B)	19.26
	(C)	19.27
	D	19.27
	(E)	19.27
19.19	A	19.28
	(B)	19.28
	(C)	19.30
	(D)	19.30
	E	19.30
19.20	A	19.33/19.34
	(B)	19.34
	(C)	19.34
	D	19.34
	(E)	19.34
19.21	A	19.34
	(B)	19.34
	(C)	19.34
	D	19.35
	(E)	19.34

19.22
(A) 19.211
(B) 19.211
C 19.211
D 19.211
(E) 19.211

19.23
(A) 19.214
(B) 19.214
(C) 19.214
D 19.214
(E) 19.214

19.24
A 19.213
B 19.214
C 19.216
D 19.215
(E) 19.217

19.25
(A) 19.231
B 19.231
C 19.231
(D) 19.231
(E) 19.231

19.26
A 19.228
(B) 19.228
(C) 19.228
(D) 19.228
E 19.228

19.27
(A) 19.229
(B) 19.229
C 19.229
D 19.229
(E) 19.229

19.28
A 19.40
(B) 19.40
C 19.40
(D) 19.40
E 19.43

19.29
A 19.47
(B) 19.48
(C) 19.49
(D) 19.50
E 19.50

19.30
(A) 19.173
(B) 19.173
(C) 19.173
(D) 19.174
(E) 19.174

19.31
(A) 19.176
(B) 19.176
C 19.176
D 19.176
(E) 19.176

19.32
A 19.183
(B) 19.183
(C) 19.184
(D) 19.184
E 19.183

19.33
(A) 19.252
(B) 19.252
C 19.252
(D) 19.252
(E) 19.254

SECTION 20: DISEASES OF THE SKIN

20.1
(A) 20.14
(B) 20.14
C 20.14
D 20.14
(E) 20.14

20.2
A 20.67
(B) 20.67
(C) 20.67
D 20.67
E 20.67

20.3
A 20.70
B 20.70
C 20.70
(D) 20.71
E 20.71

20.4
(A) 20.26
B 20.26
C 20.26
(D) 20.26
(E) 20.26

20.5
(A) 20.37
B 20.37
(C) 20.38
D 20.39
E 20.38

20.6
A 20.40
(B) 20.40
(C) 20.41
D 20.41
(E) 20.41

20.7
A 20.46
(B) 20.46
C 20.46
(D) 20.46
(E) 20.46

20.8
A 20.53
(B) 20.53
(C) 20.53
D 20.53
E 20.54

20.9
(A) 20.51
(B) 20.51
C 20.51
(D) 20.51
E 20.51

20.10
(A) 20.39
(B) 20.39
(C) 20.39
(D) 20.39
(E) 20.39

20.11
A 20.42
B 20.42
(C) 20.42
(D) 20.42
(E) 20.42

20.12
(A) 20.67
(B) 20.67
(C) 20.67
D 20.67
E 20.68

20.13	(A)	20.96	20.14	(A)	20.66	20.15	A	20.70
	B	20.96		(B)	20.81		B	20.87
	(C)	20.96		(C)	20.81		(C)	20.87
	(D)	20.96		(D)	20.81		(D)	20.87
	(E)	20.96		(E)	20.81		(E)	20.87

20.16	A	20.94
	(B)	20.94
	(C)	20.94
	D	20.94
	E	20.94

SECTION 21: NEUROLOGY

21.1	(A)	21.11	21.2	(A)	21.82	21.3	(A)	21.138
	(B)	21.11		(B)	21.83		(B)	21.93
	(C)	21.11		C	21.82		(C)	21.127
	D	21.10		(D)	21.83		(D)	21.93
	(E)	21.11		E	21.82		E	21.93

21.4	(A)	21.127	21.5	A	21.120	21.6	(A)	21.274
	(B)	22.16		B	21.120		(B)	21.274
	(C)	21.177		C	21.120		C	21.274
	D	21.212		(D)	21.120		(D)	21.274
	(E)	21.244		(E)	21.120		E	21.274

21.7	A	21.161	21.8	A	21.110	21.9	A	21.154
	(B)	21.160/21.170		(B)	21.110		(B)	21.153
	C	21.161		C	21.110		C	21.154
	D	21.161		D	21.110		D	21.154
	(E)	21.160/21.170		E	21.110		(E)	21.153

21.10	(A)	21.208	21.11	A	21.208	21.12	A	21.212
	B	21.206		(B)	21.207		(B)	21.213
	(C)	21.207		C	21.207		C	21.214
	(D)	21.209		(D)	21.207		D	21.214
	E	21.210		E	21.207		E	21.216

21.13	A	21.219	21.14	(A)	21.228	21.15	(A)	21.230
	(B)	21.219/21.220		B	21.228		(B)	21.230
	C	21.221		(C)	21.228		C	21.230
	D	21.222		D	21.228		(D)	21.230
	E	21.223		E	21.228		(E)	21.230

21.16			21.17			21.18		
	(A)	21.240		(A)	21.244		(A)	21.254
	(B)	21.240		(B)	21.244		(B)	21.254
	C	21.240		C	21.244		C	21.254
	(D)	21.240		(D)	21.244		(D)	21.254
	E	21.240		(E)	21.244		(E)	21.125

21.19			21.20			21.21		
	(A)	21.55		A	21.56		A	21.63
	(B)	21.59		(B)	21.56		B	21.63
	(C)	21.60		(C)	21.56		C	21.63
	D	21.66		(D)	21.56		(D)	21.63
	E	21.60		E	21.63		(E)	21.63

21.22		
	(A)	21.270
	(B)	21.270
	(C)	21.270
	D	21.270
	(E)	21.270

SECTION 22: DISEASES OF VOLUNTARY MUSCLE

22.1			22.2			22.3		
	A	22.7		(A)	22.11		(A)	22.16
	(B)	22.8		(B)	22.12		B	22.17
	C	22.8		(C)	22.12		(C)	22.17
	D	22.7		D	22.12		D	22.17
	E	22.9		(E)	22.12		(E)	22.16

SECTION 23: DISORDERS OF THE EYE

23.1			23.2			23.3		
	A	23.1		(A)	23.2		(A)	23.4
	(B)	23.1		(B)	23.2		B	23.4
	C	23.1		(C)	23.2		(C)	23.4
	(D)	23.1		D	23.2		D	23.5
	(E)	23.2		E	23.2		E	23.4

23.4			23.5			23.6		
	A	23.9		A	23.15		A	23.18
	B	23.9		(B)	23.15		B	23.18
	(C)	23.12		C	23.15		C	23.18
	D	23.9		(D)	23.16		D	23.18
	(E)	23.9		(E)	23.15		(E)	23.3

23.7		
	(A)	23.19
	(B)	23.18
	(C)	23.9
	D	23.18
	(E)	23.18

SECTION 24: DISORDERS OF UNCERTAIN AETIOLOGY

24.1
(A) 24.13
(B) 24.14
(C) 20.68
D 24.15
E 24.14

24.2
(A) 24.10
(B) 24.10
(C) 24.10
(D) 24.10
E 24.10

24.3
A 24.4
(B) 24.5
(C) 24.5
(D) 24.6
E 24.5

24.4
A 24.7
(B) 24.7
(C) 24.7
(D) 24.7
(E) 24.7

SECTION 25: PSYCHIATRY AND MEDICINE

25.1
(A) 25.48
B 25.10
(C) 25.48
D 25.48
(E) 25.48

25.2
A 25.22
(B) 25.22
(C) 25.22
(D) 25.22
(E) 25.22

25.3
A 25.20
(B) 25.20
(C) 25.20
(D) 25.20
(E) 25.20

25.4
A 25.49
(B) 25.48
C 25.49
(D) 25.49
(E) 25.49

25.5
(A) 25.46
B 25.46
(C) 25.47
D 25.46
(E) 25.47

25.6
A 25.16
(B) 25.16
(C) 25.16
D 25.23
E 25.23

25.7
A 25.42
B 25.42
(C) 25.42
(D) 25.42
(E) 25.42

SECTION 26: SPORTS MEDICINE

26.1
(A) 26.3
(B) 26.3
(C) 26.3
D 26.3
(E) 26.3

26.2
A 26.1
B 26.2
(C) 26.2
(D) 26.2
(E) 26.2

26.3
A 26.1
(B) 26.1
C 26.1
D 26.1
(E) No reference

26.4
(A) 26.5
B 26.6
C 26.6
D 26.6
E 26.6

26.5
(A) 26.6
(B) 26.7
(C) 26.8
(D) 26.8
E 26.5

26.6
A 26.6
(B) 26.7
(C) 26.7
D 26.7
(E) 26.7

26.7
A 26.5
B 26.5
C 26.5
(D) 26.5
(E) 26.5

SECTION 27: MEDICINE IN OLD AGE

27.1
(A) 27.9
(B) 27.9
(C) 27.9
D 27.9
E 27.9

27.2
A 27.3
B 27.3
(C) 27.3
D 27.3
(E) 27.3

SECTION 28: TERMINAL CARE

28.1
(A) 28.5
B 28.10
C 28.10
(D) 28.10
(E) 28.10

28.2
(A) 28.4
B 28.4
(C) 28.4
D 28.4
(E) 28.5

INDEX

This index contains an alphabetical listing of all the main topics included in this book. Each entry is followed by a page number and the actual question number in brackets: ie 26 (10) refers to page 26 question number 10.